The Chickens Fight Back

· · ·

PANDEMIC PANICS *and*

DEADLY DISEASES THAT JUMP

from ANIMALS TO HUMANS

· · ·

DAVID WALTNER-TOEWS

GREYSTONE BOOKS

DOUGLAS & MCINTYRE PUBLISHING GROUP

VANCOUVER/TORONTO/BERKELEY

07 08 09 10 11   5 4 3 2 1

The quote on page 41 from *The Plague,* by Albert Camus, is from a translation by
Stuart Gilbert, published by The Modern Library, Random House, 1948.

Greystone Books
A division of Douglas & McIntyre Ltd.
2323 Quebec Street, Suite 201
Vancouver, British Columbia
Canada V5T 4S7
www.greystonebooks.com

Library and Archives Canada Cataloguing in Publication
Waltner-Toews, David, 1948–
The chickens fight back : pandemic panics and deadly diseases
that jump from animals to humans / David Waltner-Toews.

Includes bibliographical references and index.
ISBN 978-1-55365-270-0

1. Epidemics. 2. Zoonoses. I. Title.
RA639.W37 2007   614.4'3   C2006-907001-6

Editing by Nancy Flight
Copy editing by Wendy Fitzgibbons
Jacket and text design by Naomi MacDougall
Jacket illustration: Heritage Image Partnership/First Light
Printed and bound in Canada by Friesens
Printed on acid-free paper that is forest friendly (100% post-consumer
recycled paper) and has been processed chlorine free.
Distributed in the U.S. by Publishers Group West

We gratefully acknowledge the financial support of the Canada Council for the Arts,
the British Columbia Arts Council, the Province of British Columbia through the Book
Publishing Tax Credit, and the Government of Canada through the Book Publishing
Industry Development Program (BPIDP) for our publishing activities.

For two great teachers of veterinary epidemiology—

the late John Iverson,

who inspired me to care about

the dead skunk in the middle of the road,

and Wayne Martin,

who taught me to measure its significance

From ghoulies and ghosties

And long-leggedy beasties

And things that go bump in the night,

Good Lord, deliver us!

Traditional Scottish Prayer

Of Pandemic Panic

And Scurrying Beasties,

Of Singing and Flight,

And Things That Go Bump in the Night,

With All Our Most Constant Companions,

Shall We Tell Our Tales of Woe and Delight.

An Epidemiologist's Fireside Rhyme

CONTENTS

. . .

And Things That Go Bump in the Night

With All Our Most Constant Companions

Shall We Tell Our Tales of Woe and Delight

Of Pandemic Panic

. . .

A BRIEF INTRODUCTION *to* THINKING

ABOUT EPIDEMICS, PANDEMICS, *and*

DISEASES PEOPLE GET *from* ANIMALS

. . .

(1)

AN IMAGE LOOKING FOR A STORY

O N TELEVISION, workers in white biohazard suits in British Columbia carry away garbage bags filled with dead chickens. A reporter's voice says not to worry. These chickens have a mild strain of the flu virus, but (the reporter says) it is not a problem for people. From ramshackle villages in Southeast Asia, eastern Europe, the Middle East, and Africa, we see images of more workers in white suits, carrying similar trash bags. They could be the same ones we saw in Canada, for all we know, and maybe even the same white-suited aliens who, in 1994, greeted possible plague-carrying travelers from India at Canadian airports. Barefoot children dash around the workers' feet, gleefully chasing chickens through the dirt to help the spacemen. Again, we are told not to worry. Everything is under control.

My heart is racing. North American and European governments stockpile drugs and vaccines. We will be okay, won't we? The stock exchanges won't collapse, will they?

As an epidemiologist, a veterinarian, and, mostly, a human being living inside the North American castle, I am both embarrassed and anxious. North American television viewers, already jittery about their safety in the world, are given numbers: this many cases in animals, this many in people. They are shown a map of wild-waterfowl migrations, the same map of hypothetical lines shown again and again, presented by medical personnel from Geneva or Washington with the serious authority of newly minted converts to ecology and evolution. Viewers are told details of viral structure in an alphanumeric code: H5N1. But there is no context, no narrative. What are they to do with this information? Like one of Oliver Sacks's patients with profound amnesia, we panic. What is going on? Why do these numbers and letters seem to mean so much to the people announcing them?

What are viewers to make of the children for whom this catching of chickens is, as all things in childhood should be, a game? What are they to make of the work-weary mothers and fathers in their farm clothes leaning in adobe and thatch and worn wooden doorways, the despair in their eyes as they see their dinners, their bank accounts, their jobs being toted away? Why are they not happy to save the world from economic collapse?

Before these questions can be answered and the sky propped back up where it belongs, avian influenza needs to be put into context. This so-called bird flu is not a unique disease. It belongs to a very large extended family of diseases that are shared among other animals and people. They are called zoonotic diseases, or "zoonoses" (pronounced zoó-uh-no-sees) for short.

All the infectious diseases people have ever cared about have come to us from other animals. These include all the big killers, such as measles, tuberculosis, and smallpox. Some made the jump to people and decided they liked our lifestyles. They liked what we ate, where we hiked, how we loved to crowd together, how we enjoyed inserting juicy appendages into each other.

Other diseases have visited us from their animal hosts fairly regularly, but really, when push comes to shove, they like their old animal homes best. These ailments still mostly live in animals and only periodically make the jump to people—rabies, for

instance, and other strange diseases with historical or popular names such as poker players' pneumonia (caused by a small,
virus-like agent), Bang's disease (caused by bacteria, usually
acquired through milk, and once called, by British troops, Malta
fever), and Dum-Dum fever (a parasitic disease also called kala-
azar, or leishmaniasis).

The ones that scare us are the microbes that make the leap
across species today, causing what are called emerging infectious diseases, as if they are somehow coming out of something,
a womb, perhaps, or a deep sleep. The agents (and scientists do
call them agents) that cause these diseases are the spies from the
animal world sent to check out human beings as possible new
hosts: the viruses that cause SARS (severe acute respiratory syndrome), avian influenza, and Nipah virus encephalitis.

One of the reasons many public health workers are anxious
is that they don't know whether these agents will become permanent residents in human bodies and populations or whether
they are just tourists, zoonoses passing through. All of us would
prefer, of course, that after a few weeks of pillaging, they return
home, like the Vikings. That possibility requires that there are
some populations of animals around for them to go back to. I
have friends who cannot go back to Yugoslavia; Yugoslavia does
not exist. And there are infectious agents that might not be able
to go back to the animal homes from whence they came, because
we are driving those natural hosts to extinction.

Many citizens of industrialized countries are also afraid
because they are surprised, shocked even, at the very idea that
infectious agents from animals can affect people. People don't
like surprises. Surprises mess up economic and political plans,
throw theories into disarray, and perplex us.

This surprise is part of a deep, collective amnesia about who
we are as a species and where we have come from. To anyone with
an elementary understanding of the long sweep of the earth's

social and ecological history, the emergence of these diseases is not surprising at all.

This book is an attempt to revive our memories and to tell our collective story in a way you have perhaps not heard before. We are surrounded by microbes, but don't let the thought of all those tiny possible disease causers out there paralyze you or drive you into a frenzy of spraying and killing. The living things on this planet are one big, dysfunctional extended family of species, in which most bacteria, viruses, and parasites are beneficial and necessary, in which diseases have a useful role in nature, and in which we ourselves have evolved from microbes and are composed of them.

I think we—this big family, including the bothersome and wonderful and contradictory human species—can work out our problems with the help of some serious narrative therapy. I don't think we need to go to war. The diseases that spring from microbial infections are controllable, sometimes even preventable. After millennia of war on disease and the eradication of some of the worst, we might even find ways to live together with a lot of infections out there, engaging in minor, stylized skirmishes, a reasonable, acceptable death toll on all sides. All it takes is a bit of biological common sense, a long-sleeved shirt, and some careful attention to this amazing planet we live on.

In the meantime, turn off the television and read this book. Brush away those mosquitoes, raise a glass of red wine, share some dark chocolate. Talk to your friends, including the animals. Sing to them, with them. Make music. We will all die. That is a normal part of life. And there are ways to make our dying more pleasant, less catastrophic, more as if we are among mortal friends. If we understand just a little more about the animals we share this planet with and the micro-organisms that they carry around, we might even begin to understand ourselves.

And that would be a tale well worth telling our grandchildren.

(2)

EPIDEMICS, PANDEMICS, AND
ZOONOSES: AN INTRODUCTION

*A*VIAN INFLUENZA, the so-called bird flu, has been described, by various people who should know these things—
spokespeople from the World Health Organization (WHO) and
the United States' Centers for Disease Control and Prevention—
as the single greatest threat facing the world. Not war, not poverty, not starvation, not catastrophic climate change. Bird flu.

Okay, let's play a bit of Bill Clinton here. What do these authorities mean by "threat"? (We should also ask what they mean by
"bird" and "flu," but that is a story for another time.) Let us begin
with "threat."

A threat, in this sense, is something that is likely to cause us
harm; we could also use the word "danger." Bird flu is the biggest danger facing the world, these authorities are saying, and to
deal with this threat, better security is needed. Until a few years
ago, we scientists had banished words like "threat" and "danger"
and reduced them to the more scientifically controllable, measur-
able word "risk." Our response to danger was called "risk management." Now, in the new age of emerging infectious diseases
such as bird flu, we seem to be back in the jungle. We are back
to dangers and threats. The worst of these, today's equivalent to

the man-eating lion in the dark forest, is a pandemic. The word "pandemic" is often bandied about in the same conversations as "threat." One of my colleagues has defined a pandemic as an epidemic, only "huger," which is as accurate a description as any.

So what is an epidemic? It is like an outbreak, only huger. An outbreak occurs when a relatively small group of people or animals or plants gets sick, as when everyone gets sick after eating a warm potato salad on a sunny day. The source of an outbreak can usually be traced to one particular event or exposure.

The word "epidemic" goes at least as far back as Homer, in about the eighth century BC. Homer used it to refer to someone in his or her own country, as differentiated from a traveler. It had connotations of "indigenous" or "endemic." Hippocrates, in 430 BC, gave it a medical slant, referring to physical syndromes (illnesses) that occurred in particular places and times. After the discovery of bacteria in the nineteenth century, people began to use the term to refer to specific diseases, as in epidemics of cholera. More recently, the word has been used to refer to more cases than expected of both very specific diseases, such as hemolytic uremic syndrome caused by *E. coli* 0157:H7, and general syndromes, such as obesity. In this book, I shall assume that an epidemic occurs when many people or animals get sick and perhaps die, usually countrywide.

A pandemic is a lot of people getting sick and dying in many countries at more or less the same time. In response to the threat of avian influenza, WHO recently updated its criteria for what it calls a pandemic. Its classification includes an Inter-Pandemic Phase (which thus assumes we are always between pandemics, as we are between ice ages), in which other animals, but no people, are infected and ranges up through various Pandemic Alert phases, in which the agents from other species are trying us out but haven't fully adapted to us, to Phase 6, the Pandemic Phase, in which there is "increased and sustained transmission in the general population." After that, waves of the disease go around the world, but fewer people get sick and die with each subsequent wave, either because humans have built up immunity or because the agent, defying creationists, evolves through the process of natural selection. In this case, only those with milder forms of the disease survive long enough to pass it on to others, and hence the agent moves in with our species to a longer, gentler, more sustainable life. Finally, through some combination of heroic efforts on our part and the natural progression of events, we arrive at another Inter-Pandemic Phase.

When we say that a lot of people are getting sick or dying, what do we mean? How many people is a lot of people? What do we mean by "sick"? Epidemiologists sometimes define an epidemic as more cases than they would expect, or as "unusually high rates" of disease or death. What is "unusual"? What is "unexpected"? How, indeed, does one measure the importance of a disease?

Each year there are several hundred million cases of malaria, and a million or so people die, mostly children. Tuberculosis kills a couple of million people a year. HIV/AIDS and AIDS-related illnesses kill millions every year. Diarrhea kills millions of children every year. Some diseases have a high case-fatality rate, meaning that a large proportion of those who get the disease die. Some of these diseases affect only a few people, and so the fatality rate in the overall population is very small. Other diseases have low case-fatality rates, but many people are infected, so the total number of people who die in the population is very high. Many global assessments by the World Health Organization, the World Bank, and other large organizations now use measures such as disability-adjusted life years (DALY) and disability-free life expectancy (DFLE) to compare the importance of various diseases. Using these measures emphasizes afflictions of children (who have more years of life to lose than older people), such as diarrhea, malaria, suicide, and accidents. These measure also give greater weight to chronic, debilitating diseases than to acute outbreaks. How do we assess importance? Is it a scientific decision?

Are authorities more hesitant to use the loaded word "pandemic" for some diseases, preferring to speak of a "global epidemic" of AIDS or "high rates" of malaria or diarrhea in certain parts of the world? If so, why is that? Do some diseases so radically and explicitly expose global economic inequities that the wealthy owners of global institutions would prefer to focus on those that more directly threaten Europe and North America and for which a technical, money-making fix is more likely to be found? The truth is that although words like "outbreak," "epidemic," and "pandemic" have a scientific ring to them, and some grounding in science, their use is very political.

I don't want to belittle the possibility of a pandemic of some sort of plague. Indeed, by the time you read this, perhaps that plague will be upon us. I just want us all to understand that, in the way we talk about and respond to diseases in the world community, we are going beyond science to make value judgments about what is unexpected or unusual. In one sense, every death is expected and tragic. Baby-boomer optimism about technological breakthroughs notwithstanding, death is, and will remain, the usual course of events. The world could not unfold as it should if we did not all, sooner or later, die. This eventuality is what gives us despair and our children hope. We have come to expect that our deaths will occur later in life, however, and by heart attacks, cancer, suicide, or car accidents (which are on the top ten world killer list), not attacks of chicken viruses, for goodness' sake.

There is a measure of poetic justice in the idea that the next global pandemic could come from chickens, that they should make us even more fearful than the explosive strutting of half-cocked fanatics that attempted to hijack the global story after 2001. We, industrial societies, have been the ones who called for a chicken in every pot. In our conquest of hunger and pursuit of obesity, we were the ones who pushed for economies of scale in agriculture, which not only brought down the consumer price of good protein but created vast brewing vats for a multitude of infectious microbes. Chickens have been on the front line of our battles against nature and hunger—and our fanatical obsession with personal health, low taxes, and the economics of me-ism. This is, then, the revenge of the pawns.

In this current avian influenza scenario, the chickens really are like pawns, since they are only the messengers from a beleaguered biosphere to cocky human beings. So far, the general response has been to shoot the messengers. If we want to stay around in a convivial world, our species shall have to do better; we shall have to come to some accommodation with the kings and queens and bishops hiding in the back row. This is not a battle to win. The best we can hope for is an uneasy, mutually respectful draw.

The flu pandemic could kill a billion people, or maybe just a few dozen. If it is a real killer, by the time we know (the viruses change so fast that we won't know until they are upon us), it will be too late to make a vaccine. By the time the vaccine would be produced, those who are going to die would already be dead. Scientists and public health workers think there is a pandemic coming, but they are not sure. No one knows which agent it will be or where it will come from. The better the detection methods become, the more precise the tests, the more refined the technology, the more viruses and other tiny living things can be seen— the less is known about what they mean.

Emerging infectious diseases such as avian influenza have created a dilemma for scientists: what we know we don't know seems to be expanding faster than what we are pretty sure we do know. We have a lot of hard facts and a poor understanding of what they mean. What kind of advice can be given to policymakers? How can scientists and politicians incorporate a sense of uncertainty and ignorance into their activities? How do we do this and still whistle while we work?

There are ways, but they are ways that many scientists and most politicians have been trying to ignore. Twenty-first-century problems cannot be solved using only nineteenth- and twentieth-century scientific methods, and there is a kind of child-like simplicity in supposing they can. Many scientific methods require us to put on blinkers and focus on small things. A lot can be learned by studying the genetics of viruses and the structure of human cells, but the questions now facing the world are bigger: Where does a pandemic come from? Can it be predicted or prevented, and, if not, what is the best way to respond and adapt? How can people live in healthy peace with nature on this planet? These questions require a combination of the best laboratory science with an understanding of ecology, culture, social change, and ethics. This is no time to put on blinkers, either running to the apocalyptic and conservative religious and economic cults that daily evangelize in the headlines or retreating to the kind of experimental laboratory science that was excellent at solving an entirely different set of problems. Humanity has come too far, learned too many good things, to make that retreat.

Avian influenza is only one of a great many zoonoses, some of which have changed the course of history and some of which circulate among us undetected—sleeper cells, perhaps, or maybe just small sleeping companions. Occasionally, in small acts of generosity, we share them back.

WHO defines zoonoses as those diseases caused by agents that are naturally transmitted between other vertebrates and humans. The late Calvin Schwabe, a zoologist, veterinarian, epidemiologist, medical anthropologist, humanist, chef, and pioneer in the study of what has been called "one medicine"—the common historical roots and substantive relationships between human and animal medicine—took a slightly more liberal view of zoonoses.

In his *Veterinary Medicine and Human Health,* he defined zoonoses as diseases whose agents are shared in nature among people and other vertebrate species. His definition thus includes not just infections transmitted from vertebrate animals to people, but also a wide array of diseases that people and other animals have in common because of environments they share, as well as diseases that occur because animals create hospitable environments for human pathogens, even though the animals may not necessarily serve as reservoirs, nor transmit the agents directly to people. Pedro Acha and Boris Szyfres, writing for the Pan American Health Organization, worked around some of these ambiguities by entitling their major text in the area *Zoonoses and Communicable Diseases Common to Man and Animals.*

Reservoirs for zoonoses are their natural home—those animals or combination of animals and ecosystems in which the infectious agents usually live and multiply and on which they depend for survival. If the reservoir is a single animal, it's called a reservoir host (which should mean, if life were fair, that we would call the microbe a guest, which we don't; we denigrate it by calling it a parasite or pathogen). Microbes usually don't kill their reservoir hosts, or, if they do, they take a while to do so, or they find ways to get themselves transmitted to another animal (through biting or contaminating the environment, for instance) before the first animal dies.

Most often, humans are "accidental" hosts of the agent (as if, in other types of diseases, we are deliberately targeted). If we are "accidental hosts," the microbe doesn't need us; we just happen to provide a handy bed-and-breakfast while it is looking for someone else. Sometimes we are a dead-end host, a kind of Hotel California, from which the agent can check out but never leave (alive, that is).

Zoonoses may be classified according to the animals that are their natural homes, such as chickens, dogs, rodents, bats, or non-human primates. This classification helps us to think carefully about the species with which we interact, how we interact with them, and how we might manage those interactions. People provide opportunities for zoonoses by creating habitats for some types of animals (raccoons and pet cats, for instance, in urban environments, or white-tailed deer and cows in North American farmland) or by invading the habitats of other animals, such as bats, wild primates, or migrating birds.

We increase the chances that an organism will jump across species when we interact more closely with those species. About four hundred free-ranging rhesus macaques live at the Swayamb-hunath Temple in Kathmandu, Nepal, interacting with residents and visitors by sharing water, food, and aggressive play. Scientists have only begun to investigate the disease risks associated with such temples, common throughout South and Southeast Asia. In North America, people play with their pet dogs and cats or take them into hospitals in animal visitation programs, raising similar questions. The stakes are raised if we engage in that most intimate contact of all—eating another species. One theory of the emergence of HIV/AIDS is that people killed and ate non-human primates from which they picked up the virus. Why people would dine thus—being marginalized, poor, and driven into the forest margins—is part of the larger story, which I hope becomes apparent as you read this book.

Zoonoses may also be classified ecologically, according to the cycles of infection that maintain them in nature and the ways they are communicated between animals and from other animals to people. Direct zoonoses, which include many food-borne agents like *Salmonella* and *E. coli* 0157:H7, may be perpetuated in nature by a single vertebrate species, such as birds or cattle; their natural cycles require no invertebrates, and they are transmitted to people directly, through bites or food. This book will not dwell on food-borne zoonoses; those diseases, including newly emerging ones such as bovine spongiform encephalopathy (mad cow disease), will be covered more thoroughly in the forthcoming second edition of my book *Food, Sex and Salmonella.*

Cyclozoonoses have maintenance cycles that require more than one vertebrate species but no invertebrates. *Echinococcus multilocularis,* a parasite found in dogs, is an example.

Metazoonoses require both vertebrates and invertebrates, such as ticks or mosquitoes, to complete the life cycle. The plague, which needs fleas, and American sleeping sickness, which requires triatomid bugs (also called kissing bugs), are metazoonotic diseases.

Finally, saprozoonoses depend on inanimate reservoirs or development sites, such as soil, water, or plants, as well as vertebrate hosts. Some of the parasitic diseases we get from our pets, like toxoplasmosis and toxocariasis, require an external environment to complete their life cycles; their eggs do not become infectious for another animal until they have "ripened" in the environment for days to weeks.

Other saprozoonoses, which aren't zoonoses by the WHO definition, grow in the environment, from which they make people and other animals sick. In 2001, for instance, dogs, cats, harbor seals, porpoises, ferrets, llamas, and people in and around a particular area of Vancouver Island all suffered serious lung and neurological infections from an environmental fungus called *Cryptococcus gattii.* Interestingly, the strain of the fungus that caused the outbreak usually lives in the tropics and subtropics. Some people suggested climate change might have contributed to its spread. This book does not dwell on such diseases but focuses on diseases we get *from* animals rather than those we get *with* animals.

To the classifications above, laboratory scientists would add a system differentiated according to bacterium, virus, and parasite species. In this book, I have used a variation on the ecological and animal-reservoir themes. It has a separate section for each of the following types of zoonoses: those that involve insects and a variety of other animals, but no birds ("And Scurrying Beasties"); those that involve birds, with or without insects ("Of Singing and Flight"); those that involve rats and bats ("And Things That Go Bump in the Night"); and those that involve animals that we have domesticated and with which we have evolved especially close relationships ("With All Our Most Constant Companions"). It is thus a hybrid classification system based on animal reservoirs, natural cycles, and the relationships of the animal reservoirs to people. It seemed to me to best reflect how intelligent non-scientists might classify them and begin to make sense of them.

Some zoonoses have been around for a long time and will be for millennia to come; our species should live so long. Microbes of all sorts, all those microscopic "animalcules" that the Dutch scientist Anton van Leeuwenhoek first saw through his microscope in the late 1600s, are all around us, in our mouths, on our genitals, on our hands. And certainly all over those other animals with which we share the planet. Your dog could be carrying them, or your cat, or the mosquitoes zinging around your ear as you read this book on the veranda in the evening; they could be in your salad or in those cute raccoons waddling across the backyard. The diseases caused by these microbes have names that are both familiar and odd and include the plague, West Nile virus infection, Lyme disease, sleeping sickness, salmonellosis, poker players' pneumonia, and tuberculosis. These diseases can—and do—strike many people every day. They show up as worms in the eye and cysts in the belly, chronic heart disease, and debilitating infections of the brain.

Usually zoonoses drive through our neighborhoods and check us out without our even knowing. We then, as some researchers have said, "suffer" from subclinical disease. Not every infection (when the bug gets into you and multiplies) results in clinical disease. Sometimes these infections do kill. Most often they cause a passing, "flu-like" illness.

The more perceptive among my readers will have noticed a little trick I have been playing in the last few paragraphs. I have been slipping back and forth between diseases and infections, and between animals and people. When we speak of pandemics of diseases people get from animals, we need to be more careful. It is possible to have a pandemic infection in animals or people without a lot of disease. Infection does not equal disease. Infection in animals does not equal disease in people. Thus, we would prefer that if there is a pandemic, it be a pandemic of infection in animals (which avian influenza already is), or at least a pandemic disease in birds (which it already is), but not a pandemic disease in people.

Some writers differentiate these by using the terms "epizootic" and "panzootic" to refer to epidemics and pandemics in animals other than people. Although this usage simplifies some things for bureaucrats and managers, it obscures the fact that people are animals—exceptional animals, to be sure, but animals nonetheless—and that the sharing of microbes among species is normal. The "——demic" and "——zootic" allows people to fall back too readily into a kind of delusional silo mentality. No realistic understanding of zoonoses and their control can be achieved without the contributions of natural scientists (ecologists, entomologists, and zoologists, for instance), health scientists (veterinarians and physicians), historians, anthropologists, social scientists, artists, and just plain folks.

The bad news is that many of the threats of disease we face today are connected to each other—and to many of the things we have come to cherish in our modern lifestyles. The way we deal with one disease, or even one so-called problem, can have far-flung consequences for what happens to other diseases and other problems. The good news equally is that many of the threats of disease we face today are connected to each other—and to many of the things we have come to cherish in our modern lifestyles. The way that one disease or problem is dealt with can have far-flung consequences for what happens to other diseases and other problems. As Douglas Adams realized when he wrote *The Hitch-hiker's Guide to the Galaxy,* the answer to the question of "life, the universe and everything else" is relatively simple and hard to get our heads—and our lives—around. It may not be "42," as the computer in the novel suggests, but it is not necessarily billions of dollars of better biomedical technology and vaccines, as others propose. Some of our other options will become apparent in the tales in the book.

Let us begin, then. And what better way to begin than with the plague.

And Scurrying Beasties

• • •

DISEASES PEOPLE GET *from* ANIMALS,

INVOLVING MAMMALS *and* ARTHROPODS

(INSECTS *and* ARACHNIDS), *but* NOT BIRDS

• • •

(3)

PLAGUES, RATS, AND

THE PERFECTION OF FLEAS

*A*CCORDING TO the singer and songwriter Leonard Cohen, "everybody knows" that a plague is coming. If they don't know, then Laurie Garrett can quickly set them straight; the journalist penned *The Coming Plague,* the remarkable tome about the adventurer-scientists who have investigated infectious diseases over the past century. If there is not a plague on all our houses, there is at least a plague in every neighborhood. If you google "plague," or even restrict yourself to a more scholarly search of references to "plague," you will turn up not just the Black Death (which was probably caused by the bacterium *Yersinia pestis*) and the white plague, but also the plague monkeys, the forgotten plague, the slow plague, the Bombay plague, the ocean plague, duck plague, fowl plague, swine plague, mosquito plague, a plague of sheep, of cattle, of insects, of censorship, the plague year, plague days, plague dogs, and the Nevada mouse plague. Tracing its origins back to a Greek word for misfortune or blow, the word "plague" has been attached to just about anything that people fear or don't like.

This widespread usage of the word "plague" in our society goes deep to a wound in our cultural psyche. None of these plagues, however, are actually *the* plague, the disease associated with the bacterium *Yersinia pestis* that in 1994 so terrorized the world that between 200,000 and 300,000 people fled Surat, India, before the rumors of their worst fears, and startled North American television viewers were faced with the sight of white-masked officials inspecting passengers arriving from India at our airports.

People's fears of the plague are not without foundation. Beginning with the Justinian plague (AD 541–544) in Egypt, the plague crested around the world in at least three major pandemics and is at least partly responsible for pushing European history in new, unexpected directions. For instance, the second pandemic, the Black Death, killed off at least a third of medieval Europe—tens of millions of people—in just a few years in the mid-fourteenth century, even as it killed tens of millions of people in Asia and the Middle East. Economic and cultural changes, including peasants' revolts, the rise of capitalism, and a loss of power by the church, all happened in its wake.

That story, and the horrors and wonders associated with it, has been recounted many times and should be essential reading for any thoughtful person in the twenty-first century. All the lessons about ecology, public health, personal hygiene, climate change, compassion, fate, and the dangers of globalization that anyone would wish to learn are there, plain for those who wish to see. This statement is also true for the story of the white plague, which is actually tuberculosis, another disease of animal origin discussed more fully elsewhere in this volume (and not to be confused with another white plague, which bleaches coral reefs).

The third plague pandemic started in China in 1855 and from there was disseminated around the world. Between 1898 and 1918, more than 12 million people in India died of plague. When the pandemic subsided, like a great flood it left small, stable pools of infection cycling among rodents, fleas, and the occasional unwary person in uneasy neighborliness on every continent except Australia. In the 1990s, about a dozen countries reported outbreaks of the plague. Most outbreaks occurred in African countries such as Madagascar, Mozambique, and Tanzania, but cases were also reported from Brazil, Ecuador, Peru, Mongolia, Vietnam, China, and the United States. In 1997, an outbreak of pharyngeal (infection at the back of the throat) plague, associated with eating raw camel meat, was reported from Jordan.

The plague is a disease of increasing concern because of the growth of urban slums globally and the unstable weather conditions associated with global warming and El Niño; these lead to changes in habitat for rodents in the countryside and explosions in rodent population in urban centers. We tend to view this disease as one that affects people, which, of course, it does. But we may learn something by taking a broader view. The plague is a disease of people, of fleas, of rodents, and, finally, of whole social-ecological systems.

In people, it comes in three forms: bubonic, pneumonic, and septicemic. To cause disease, the causative organism, *Yersinia pestis*, needs to get into the bloodstream, through an open wound, through transmission from one's afflicted cat (say, by kissing the cat and inhaling the bug), or through a bite from an infected flea that then vomits the bacterium into the bloodstream. Much like the first European invaders feeding off the bounty of the American continents, once in the bloodstream the bacterium travels down the lymph rivers and bloodways, looking for appropriate places to settle and multiply. Peripheral lymph nodes—in the armpits or crotch—seem to be as good a place as any. These nodes swell painfully, and the infected person begins to feel some combination of fever, chills, headache, diarrhea, and constipation, moving on to generalized pain, rapid heartbeat, anxiety (understandably), staggering gait, slurred speech, and prostration. If untreated, 25 to 60 percent of people die. This bubonic form of plague cannot be transmitted from one person to another; an epidemic of bubonic plague depends on the continued presence of rodents and fleas. It is thus a true zoonosis.

In some people the infection moves to the lungs, where it causes pneumonia, which is a kind of adaptation of the organism to modern human society. Once in the lungs, it can be coughed out into the air and transmitted from person to person. Fleas and rats are no longer necessary. This form of the disease is called pneumonic plague. Now, or so conventional wisdom (recently called into question) has it, the bug can cause a serious epidemic or pandemic.

Although both bubonic and pneumonic plague can kill, they don't kill everyone. At least some bodies are able to fight the disease off, and people recover. In some cases, both these forms of the disease lead to a full-blown septicemic (that is, blood-borne) form, in which people develop nervous and cerebral symptoms very quickly. Pretty well all of these people die.

But the plague is not just a disease of people. It is also a disease of fleas, which are themselves something of a wonder and worthy of a small aside here. In the history and mythology of the Judeo-Christian tradition, three and seven are two numbers used to express perfection. The third perfect number in Judeo-Christian stories is forty, which is the number of days Jesus spent in the desert, and which is an excellent age to have been, but which is not relevant to the life of fleas. The flea, aside from never experiencing the joy of reaching that pinnacle of the roller-coaster of life, the fortieth birthday, is a perfect parasite.

Besides being perfect, which in and of itself is annoying, fleas are exceedingly small. They have caused me to quarrel with my wife, whom I accused, no doubt falsely, of hallucinating tiny jumping, biting specks. They are brown, wingless animals with Twiggy-like bodies that can make them seem to disappear when they face you head-on, or more likely, rear-on, and that enable them to slip unpunished into cracks and cleavages. Suctorial mouthparts, eyes, antennae, and combs bedeck the chitinous head, giving them, under the microscope, the warrior-like appearance of a military beast from a planet in the Star Wars galaxy. The thorax is divided into three, which is another sign that the Creator, as one entomologist has said, had an inordinate love of insects. From each segment of the thorax extends a pair of powerful, claw-tipped limbs. If fleas, says a scribble in the margins of my parasitology notes from my student days, were the size of people, they could jump over tall buildings. More relevant to me is the fact that fleas the size of fleas can jump from the pillow on the couch to the base of my ear.

If one were to go to the flea for moral lessons, one could learn that if it drinks enough (blood) and copulates with sufficient frequency, even a small creature can have a significant impact on the world. For those who equate "good" with "natural" and "natural" with all those living things that aren't us (a strange and pernicious equation), this may be a startling insight. Under the right conditions of decadence, a female flea, which lays from three eggs to some much larger number (probably a multiple of three) at a time, can put out a hundred of the glistening-white little things in a one-year lifetime. Fleas will lay more eggs when it is warm and the humidity is 70 percent or more. The adults live on warm-blooded animals and eggs are laid on the animals, but many of them fall off into rugs and carpets, where, like jelly beans and chocolate eggs left unfound under the sofa cushion on Easter morning, they will hatch in two to twelve days (the median of which is seven).

The yellowish-white, bristling worms—teenagers of the insect world—feed on adult flea feces (full of dried blood) hiding out in the carpets and pet-resting places where they were dropped off. They are graced with anal struts, the flea version of tight jeans. Whereas people use their struts to unhinge each other's psyches, the flea larval struts are hooks used to propel them in search of the ultimate hamburger (fecal blood casts from the adults) to stuff into their chewing mouthparts. They feed, grow, and molt three times, a process that can take anywhere from nine (three times three, under perfect conditions) to two hundred (or maybe two hundred and forty-three, which is a multiple of three) days. After the third molt, the larva spins a small cocoon, within which, like a most excellent pupil of the natural order, it pupates from seven days (under perfect conditions) to one year (usually two to four weeks, the median of which is three), after which the now-mature adult flea breaks out, seeking a host on which to feed.

In flea heaven, which has on occasion been situated on our couch, the entire life cycle takes three weeks. But fleas are quite willing to accommodate themselves to our imperfections and will stretch the process out, if they must, to two years.

There are about three thousand species and subspecies of fleas, of which only a few infest us and our pets. *Pulex irritans*, the human flea, moves freely between dogs and people, especially in the southern United States. This flea can transmit murine (mouse-related) typhus, which has less catastrophic effects than epidemic typhus, which is transmitted from rats to people by lice and has caused massive suffering and death worldwide. Epidemic typhus has been the subject of one of the classic biographies of a disease, *Rats, Lice and History*, by Hans Zinsser, which should be in every intelligent person's library.

Ctenocephalides felis (the cat flea) and *Ctenocephalides canis* (the dog flea) infest dogs, cats, and people in a kind of natural free-trade zone, although the tapeworms that they sometimes smuggle across the borders only make a home in dogs. The cat flea is probably the most common flea infesting North Americans and is the most difficult to get rid of. *Echidnophaga gallinacea*, the sticktight flea of poultry, is God's punishment for wayward dogs, cats, and young children (myself, many years ago, included) who decide to check out the inside of the chicken coop. In cats and dogs, this flea digs into the sparsely haired regions around the eyes, between the toes, and around the ears; in people, it just looks for uncovered, hairless areas.

Until relatively recently, there were few good remedies for getting rid of fleas, which spawned a huge industry in equally (in)effective treatments. Substances that effectively killed adult fleas (apart from the suffocating effects of baths) were toxic not only to fleas but also, because we share the animal kingdom with them, to us and to our pets. A California company proposed sealing off and heat-treating houses to get rid of insect infestations; this kind of drastic solution should be implemented just after first frost, in those parts of the country that get a first frost.

Other remedies for fleas proposed by several authors include: feeding the afflicted animal brewer's yeast (a teaspoon daily for a cat, a tablespoon for a fifty-pound dog), and garlic (one or two cloves per day); regularly bathing the animal with non-toxic shampoos (to suffocate the fleas), followed by a good brushing; and rubbing the dog or cat with eucalyptus oil in water and/or brewer's yeast, especially over the back around the base of the tail and in the neck area. Because treatments of afflicted animals kill only the few fleas unlucky enough to drown or get squished, baths and powders should be applied outside, where the fleas do not have the opportunity to escape into your carpet or couch. The standard veterinary literature reports that no controlled trials have demonstrated that these proposed treatments are effective. Even the herbal-treatment guru Juliette de Bairacli Levy somewhat despairingly admits that her protective lotion against ticks and lice, containing wormwood, beer, and vodka (a combination that would have a profound effect on many of us) does not affect the spartan flea.

In recent years, various hormonal remedies that interrupt larval development, combined with drugs that kill the adults, seem to be effective and safe. Removing fleas from your pet and discouraging them from reinfesting is only symptomatic treatment, however, and may aggravate the problem. Remember that many of the eggs and larvae are just hanging around the house, waiting for you to sit down. Cat fleas in particular are not fussy eaters, and, unless your whole family is on brewer's yeast, garlic, and eucalyptus baths, sitting on the couch may become a bloodbath. If you are truly serious about fleas, you must remember that though you treat your dogs or cats with baths and powders, though you deck them in eucalyptus collars and feed them garlic, brewer's yeast, or thiamine, yea, even though you spray them with the most powerful toxins, causing them to suffer even to the point of death, and treat not the couch and the rug, what you have done may not bring you to flea-free heaven.

Cat and dog fleas, so I am told, do not live well at altitudes higher than five thousand feet, so if you find that you cannot live with fleas, and you cannot, for reasons of conscience, live without them, you should lift your eyes to the hills. Know also, however, that even if you escape to Nepal or Tibet or Colorado, the tiny rat flea, *Leptopsylla segnis,* survivor in cold, dry climes, may await you there. There are fleas living on every continent, including Antarctica. Someone found a 200-million-year-old fossil flea in Australia.

There is no escape from the perfection of nature. It has predated us and shall outlive us. The religious among us might wonder if the creator invented the plague to make fleas sick and die and if we are the accidental hosts. If so, then getting rid of the plague may only encourage fleas.

Which brings us back to the plague.

Scientists suspect that *Yersinia pestis,* through one genetic mutation, adapted itself to transmission by flea bites thousands of years ago. Its cousin *Yersinia pseudotuberculosis,* which lives in rats and pigs and causes appendicitis-like food-borne illness in people, never made this adaptation. Fleas pick up *Yersinia pestis* from the blood of infected animals; the bacteria then multiply in the flea's stomach until its upper gut (proventriculus) is blocked up. Really hungry and sick to the stomach, the flea heads out to a local blood bar, ready to feed on anything—your leg, a dog's tail, a rat's butt. After taking in a huge gulp of blood, the flea regurgitates some of the bacteria back into the glass (that is, the wound on your leg), then takes a crap into it and heads on home.

A lot of fleas probably feel miserable at getting this food-borne disease (the hamburger disease of the flea world), and some of them die. Even people who love all living things usually don't care much about the personal sufferings of fleas, real or imagined, however, and no therapies have been developed to treat them and make them feel better. Penicillin would work, if one could devise a way to deliver the drug. As a veterinarian, I have had enough trouble trying to inject skinny cats and those small, nervous, snappy, skin-and-bone dogs without trying to imagine how one might inject a flea. Still, the nanotech people, I am sure, could find a way, should we decide to be more generous to other species than our reputation would suggest. One might also try anti-depressants, since they have worked in a wide range of other species; it wouldn't cure them, but they would feel better while they died, which is, I suppose, the best most of us can hope for anyway.

If fleas are bearers of bad plague news, then our warm-blooded relatives the rodents are the poor suckers who have fed and housed them all these many years. Fleas had to wait a long time before getting a good meal of rat's blood; rodents seem to have appeared on the planet some tens of millions of years ago, probably somewhere in Asia. Rats are even more recent. They appeared a few million years ago. *Yersinia pestis* causes in small rodents diseases similar to those in people, dogs, and cats. Wild rodents seem to be more resistant to the plague than domestic rodents, although plague has been known to cause major epidemics and die-offs in prairie dogs and other rural rodent cousins. Rats can carry a wide variety of diseases that can be transmitted to people, including plague, leptospirosis, typhus, spotted fever, tularemia, salmonellosis, and hantaviruses. I'll come back to some of these a bit later.

According to Hans Zinsser in *Rats, Lice and History,* black rats (*Rattus rattus*) arrived in Europe from the Far East sometime between AD 400 and AD 100. They may have been fleeing the brown rats (*Rattus norvegicus*) that ruled Asia. They may have meant to warn the Europeans about their brown relatives. The Europeans didn't listen. The so-called Norwegian rats (*Rattus norvegicus,* carried to Europe on Norwegian boats) followed from northern or northeastern China about a millennium after the black rats and pretty well wiped out their cousins.

Norway rats are Darwinian wonders, following and adapting to human habitats and adopting human behaviors with a vengeance. They reproduce with biblical perfection—about seven litters a year with seven pups per litter (well, with variance around those numbers)—and the females can breed eighteen hours after giving birth. This fecundity enables them to bounce back quickly from disease, pestilence, and human attacks. They are omnivorous and have been known to eat a third of their weight (another good biblical number) daily, voraciously consuming garbage, soap, candy, fruits, grains, seeds, and other animals, including each other. They live to be about three years old, so they live fast. They kill anything that gets in their way. They have studied us well, and bettered us.

Having been born in the Chinese Year of the Rat, I confess to having some empathy for the creatures, despite my Mennonite non-violence. My empathy does not extend so far, however, as the case described to me by a colleague who, having just returned from Tanzania, was called upon to perform some eighty dollars worth of medical and surgical procedures on an urban pet rat.

Rats are intended to have honest, hard-working lives in neighborhoods other than my own.

No one knows how many rats there are in the world, although it would not be wildly outrageous to say that there are as many of them as there are of us. Although we are never, it seems, far from rodents, most residents of North America and Europe have had few encounters with them. Growing up in a clean prairie Canadian city, I never had much to do with rodents. Reports in 1998 of rats rampaging through Chinese cities, unhindered by feral cats and dogs, chewing through garments of hotel guests and damaging power lines, do not ring any bells from my own childhood. I imagine that if such events had happened, I would have suppressed the memory so deeply that only radical psychotherapy could retrieve it.

I once caught a mouse as it shambled along the street, close to the curb. It was Sunday morning, after church, and the sun was hot: a usual Winnipeg summer Sunday. The mouse, resisting my evangelical Mennonite attentions, bit my finger when I grabbed its tail. My parents, if I remember rightly, took me to a doctor. There was some concern about tetanus. Nobody mentioned diseases such as plague or hantavirus pulmonary syndrome (see chapter 11), although we now know the agents that cause them are present in western Canadian rodents. And once, when we came home from Sunday evening church services, I remember a lot of squealing and excitement in our family; there was a mouse in the mousetrap in the front hall. The concern in this case, I think, was about protecting our food supplies.

In the southwestern United States, ground squirrels can carry the plague, which has made for some exciting, if maudlin, made-for-television movies. In 2006, a woman in Los Angeles picked up bubonic plague from an unknown source, probably a flea that jumped from rodent to cat to person. The occasional cat has passed the disease directly to an affectionately stupid person by rubbing noses.

I suppose if I had grown up on a prairie farm, I might have learned about plagues of gophers. In this case, the gophers themselves were the plague, wreaking their damage on fields. Once, in high school, I went out to Eddy Wall's farm, and we walked around with twenty-two-caliber rifles and looked for gophers to shoot. I don't remember seeing any, though I shot a few tin cans off a fence post. At that time, no one knew that small prairie rodents around the world carry dozens of different kinds of bacteria, some of which (*Bartonella* species) have, on rare occasions, infected people and caused fevers or heart problems.

My first serious encounter with rodents was in Bihar, India. At nineteen years of age, I had hitchhiked overland from Europe to Nepal and India, where I worked as a young, idealistic volunteer. Actually, that is a romantic oversimplification; running out of money in Calcutta, stunned by the poverty there and my lack of money, I had talked my way into a temporary job with the Mennonite Central Committee, helping with grain storage and distribution in a grain-for-work program to build earthen dams and improve agricultural production.

My first day in Bihar, I slept on the floor of a bookshop, and some rats brushed against my cheek in the night. Several months later, I was part of a team effort to round up rats from a grain storage building; somebody made a lot of noise behind the stacks of grain sacks, and the rest of us waited for the rats to come out. We were supposed to kill them. One rat (the only one I remember, though I know there were a lot of them) came running out and skittered up the wide pant leg of one of the Indian workers, over the crotch, and down the other leg. At least, that was the story. Lots of excitement about possible theft of the family jewels, but no talk of plague.

I don't remember our killing any rats at all; I wonder in retrospect whether our Indian co-workers, coming from a culture in which many of their compatriots feed and worship rats as companions of the god Ganesh, were just putting on a charade for the benefit of squeamish (and wealthy) westerners. They could have tried to explain things to us, but we, whose competitive and jealous God has no animal companions, would not have understood. Better to let us play our little games. Before I left Bihar, I acquired a pet chipmunk (another potential plague carrier), which I hauled around in my pocket and which ran up and down my arm to get snacks out of the palm of my hand. He later died after being accidentally locked in a refrigerator.

I tell you these stories not because I expect you to be interested in my experiences with rodents but because they indicate how far removed many of us in the industrialized world have become from the terrors of the Black Death. Yet the world would be a very different place if the plague had not turned Europe into a post-nuclear-like disaster area in the mid-fourteenth century. We are children of the plague not just in our language but also in many of our public institutions and political ideas: the collapse of feudalism, so I understand from historians, owed more to the deaths of farm laborers from the plague than it did to our enlightened moral progress as a species. And this collapse of feudalism in western Europe led to the rise of the middle class, capitalism, shopping malls, and Christian evangelical consumer cults.

Although most people think of the plague as a disease of people, and some of us (veterinarians) consider its effects on other animals, few of us think about the fact that the plague is also, perhaps most accurately, a disease of socio-ecological systems.

The Black Death occurred because the Mongol Empire had created a network for transport of goods, services, military technology, rats, fleas, and bacteria from central Asia to the gates of Europe. The Black Death occurred because Europeans, responding to longer summers and shorter winters between 700 and 1250, tripled their population, exhausted their agricultural lands, and were unprepared to adapt to the mini–ice age that followed. The Black Death occurred because prevailing winds changed, making Europe wetter—and central Asia drier—than it had been for a few hundred years. Mongol and Turk nomads, herding their flocks and joined by marmots, susliks, and other types of wild rodents, headed east and west in search of greener pastures. Europeans starved to death by the millions before the plague reached them, and those who survived the famines were weakened when the plague arrived. In this version of the narrative, *Yersinia pestis* may not even be important.

One author has suggested that the clinical signs and recurrent epidemics of the Black Death in Europe were more likely anthrax—another fatal disease people share with animals—than plague. Between outbreaks, anthrax can survive in spore form for decades and perhaps centuries in the soil (or in laboratories, but that's a different story). What is important in this narrative is that the bacteria that killed individuals were opportunists taking advantage of climatic, environmental, socio-political, and economic changes. If the plague bacteria hadn't done the job of killing, some other organisms would have; there are always plenty of candidates. And this is true for many human diseases: the specific agents (bacteria, viruses, prions) are less important than the hospitable contexts people create for them.

In 1993, a severe earthquake rattled parts of central India, damaging rodent habitats and resulting in an explosive emigration of rats from their own neighborhoods into nearby villages, where damaged grain storage facilities provided easy food and shelter. Wild rodents, under normal conditions of easy country life, may carry *Yersinia pestis* without getting sick. This phenomenon is not usually true of city rats or of rats living under crowded slum conditions. One could make a political lesson from this, but it seems too obvious.

About a year later, in August 1994, some people noticed a die-off in the rat population; after thirty years of no reported cases in India, the plague had arrived. Within weeks, some eighty cases of bubonic plague in people were reported. Since bubonic plague isn't transferred from person to person, health authorities treated the sick people and sprayed infested houses. Nobody died.

In late September, cases of pneumonic plague, which can be transmitted from person to person, showed up in Surat, a city of 1.4 million to the northwest of the original outbreak. When these cases were reported, more than 200,000 people headed out of town, and the plague became world news, with images of airport officials in Europe and North America wearing face masks and carefully screening airplanes from India. This was pandemic fear before SARS and avian influenza. But the pandemic never materialized. Some public health officials now wonder if the disease was plague at all.

Outbreaks of pneumonic plague among miners in the Democratic Republic of the Congo in 2005 and again in 2006 sickened thousands and killed hundreds, but they did not presage a pandemic explosion, as some had feared they would. Some scientists began to have second thoughts. Had *Yersinia pestis* changed its genetic colors? Were nutritional status and living conditions in the twentieth century, even at their worst, far better than living conditions a hundred years ago?

In Uganda, in 2004, a policeman from the West Nile region (ah, that cradle of Caucasians' darkest fears) called a physician, who called staff from the Centers for Disease Control and Prevention in Atlanta who happened to be in the area for a field trial on treating the plague. They found that two people had come down with pneumonic plague, and despite many human contacts, only two others—their closest caregivers—picked it up from them. You had to be close enough to get sprayed by the coughing. So, people with pneumonic plague should stay off the stage at Stratford (a prime center of spraying others with well-articulated Shakespeare). But maybe our fears are larger than the threat. Fear of our own stories, our own perceived history, casts a long shadow across our cultures.

Several years ago, one of my colleagues, an anthropologist involved in international research, came to me with a problem. "Listen," she said, "I'm working with some very dedicated scientists in a part of the world where plague has become endemic. Take a look at these reports, which concern one particular village. You're the ecosystem health expert. What should these people do?"

From the unofficial research project reports she handed to me, and a review of two decades' worth of peer-reviewed literature, I pieced together the following story:

About a century ago, the plague arrived in an area of what is now Tanzania along the trade routes and became established in several parts of the country, but not in one particular village and its environs. Then, several decades ago, the inhabitants of this village were plagued with an explosion of the rodent population, but without the occurrence of the plague. Nevertheless, the damage from the rats was sufficient to require the intervention of a special healer, who, in the manner of any good epidemiologist, intervened when the epidemic was at its peak and thus would decrease no matter what he did.

A couple of decades later, the rat plague returned, this time carrying human disease with it. Local people consulted the healer, who, it turns out, had not been paid the last time; after receiving appropriate apologies and offerings, he again suggested some cures. This time, however, perhaps because the people didn't believe hard enough or do exactly the right things, the plague persisted. Over the decade of the 1980s, thousands of people became sick, and hundreds died.

In the meantime, veterinary scientists were trapping rats and taking blood and fleas from a random sample of people and dogs, looking for *Yersinia pestis* or antibodies to it. Every possible preventive action seemed to have been tried, but nothing worked, at least not very well. Some research suggested that dogs were carrying the disease; maybe if they got rid of the dogs? An anthropologist was sent in to talk to the people to see if he could determine why nothing seemed to work.

A complicated picture emerged from the anthropologist's report, including what had been tried and why it hadn't worked.

Doctors tried to quarantine sick people, but the patients resented this intrusion into their daily lives. Under quarantine, they were prevented from leaving their homes or villages to take part in agricultural activities, gather food, care for sick relatives, or attend special occasions; some people could find loopholes, however, especially through bribery. In any case, if rat fleas were carrying the disease, it was not clear that quarantine would have any effect besides making it look as if something were being done.

One could fall back on simply diagnosing and treating cases as they came up. Since the plague is generally treatable with inexpensive antibiotics such as tetracycline or streptomycin, this approach is often the most cost-effective for sporadic (non-epidemic) cases of the plague. Treating people quickly is dependent on local treatment centers that are accessible, well staffed, and stocked with antibiotics, however. In Tanzania, the local treatment centers were accessible but not always stocked with drugs; patient records were sometimes mixed up, lost, or leaked beyond the center, raising questions of confidentiality. Patients were to bring their own bedsheets and the like; some could not do so and were ashamed of their poverty.

In many parts of the world, diagnoses are made by playing the odds. "If you hear hoofbeats," our professors at veterinary school in Saskatchewan used to say, "think horses, not zebras." But that advice needs to be taken in context. In Kenya, you might well think "zebra" at the sound of hoofbeats. In North America, we often call a fever together with either respiratory or gut problems the flu; but often it's not influenza (especially the gut form, since influenza in people is usually a respiratory disease). Sometimes that doesn't matter; "flu-like" illnesses in North America are often caused by viruses, and doctors usually treat "flu-like" viral diseases similarly (chicken soup and bed rest). In parts of Africa where the plague is known to be endemic, a lot of non-plague diseases are called the plague, including malaria. Unfortunately, malaria is not treatable by antibiotics. If only some forms of the plague, broadly interpreted as any general illness, responded to antibiotic treatment, then what advantage did those modern methods have over traditional healing?

Public health authorities tried pesticide spraying and rat poisoning in houses. People from households that had been sprayed were asked to shut all windows and doors for six hours, as well as not to clean house for three to six days. Those householders did not like to share a dwelling with dead rats and fleas for that amount of time. Moreover, the pesticides had good market value and were either allocated according to favoritism or resold to farmers as treatments for crops and foodstuffs. Some people complained of becoming ill after spraying; chickens sometimes died, and cattle became ill.

Authorities proposed that villagers plaster and seal their houses so that the rats couldn't get in from outside. Most of this work was supposed to done by women and by children under twelve, who were the ones getting sick and who did not have the energy for house renovations. Besides, there was a shortage of water needed for plastering, and men controlled the money that would pay for plastering. It was not done.

Households could move food storage outside so that the rats wouldn't come into the house: traditionally, the maize was stored outside the house. However, a decline in maize production associated with an increase in cash crop production related to an opening of world markets made maize more valuable as a tradable commodity; this development, together with a decrease in social trust (related in part to competitiveness and modernization), increased the need for vigilance. Hence the maize was now stored in the wooden ceiling of the house. Rats followed the maize into the house; this move made the dogs happy to stay around the house as well.

Public health officials recommended that householders clear shrubs and bushes from around the houses and field crops so that rats would have fewer places to hide. But arable land was scarce, and people wanted to maximize land use by planting very close to the house. Borders of fields were planted with trees to prevent soil erosion, with grasses as cattle feed, and with medicinal plants for household use. These practices were encouraged by some government agencies (obviously not those involved in eradicating the plague) to conserve soil and water. Some shrubbery was also maintained as a link to family ancestors, who were believed to live in the shrubs near the house.

Even something as apparently simple as removing food scraps from near dwellings was a problem, since this organic "waste" was thrown into the fields around the house to serve as fertilizer for the crops.

Since women and young girls prepared the food, they were getting the plague. Since children played with dogs that were infected by fleas from rats, they also got the plague.

What should these people do? To keep up agricultural production and prevent soil erosion, farmers should plant bushes and shrubs around their houses and fields. To prevent the plague, they should pull them up. To make more money, they should plant more cash crops. To bring down the price of local food, they should plant more maize. To improve their health, they should cooperate with their neighbors and move their grain into outside storehouses. To become more competitively efficient in the global market, they should compete with their neighbors. How could they decide the right path? Was there a scientific answer?

When I recounted this scenario to Jerry Ravetz, a philosopher of science and a colleague, he suggested (not without some satisfaction, I think, since philosophers, like mathematicians and theologians, seem to thrive on insoluble problems) that there might be no solution to the plague problem in Tanzania. We were up against irreducible complexity.

One might also, on a world scale, say we were up against some major cognitive dissonance. When I became a veterinarian, I was introduced to the idea that rats are intelligent, friendly, social animals that make ideal pets, especially for children. They can do tricks. Hence the eighty-dollar vet bill for the rat I mentioned earlier. Personally, I get a headache trying to reconcile rat worship, rat companionship, and the ravages of the plague. One might suggest that we have need of a kind of eco-narrative therapy for our dysfunctional species, but where would we begin?

Clearly the plague, once the terror of Europe, is no longer the killer that it once was. What did Europeans do correctly that the Tanzanian villagers can learn from?

For one thing, it has become clear that no single perspective (environmental, public health, economic, male, female) or scale (animal, household, region, world) will give us the whole picture or, if there is one, the whole solution. If the plague is seen to be a disease of individuals caused by *Yersinia pestis,* then the treatment is an antibiotic, and the delivery of disease care is where time and effort should be focused; better diagnostic laboratories need to give people greater confidence that they are being treated by the right drug for the right disease. If the plague is viewed as a disease of household dogs, rats, and fleas, then efforts should target controlling dogs, spraying for fleas, killing rats, and making sure that people have better housing. Land use planners and ecologists can monitor ecological change and target interventions when they are likely to have the greatest effects. These measures, too, are important.

Yet none of them worked in this village, because the plague is also a disease of socio-ecological systems. The price of maize, the national debt, relations between men and women in the household, the sense of neighborliness between households all need to be considered. Addressing these issues requires not just medical and technical expertise but also a deep cultural engagement and a democratic debate about trade-offs: what kind of a society do we want to live in?

Similarly, outbreaks of the plague in Mexico, Peru, Madagascar, and other countries in the 1990s could be attributed to a mix of bacterial nests left over in various landscapes from the pandemic a hundred years earlier, as well as to a lack of public health infrastructure (reflecting government spending priorities, which often reflect the muddle-headed priorities in the World Bank and the International Monetary Fund) and to cyclic meteorological events (El Niño), which have been intensified by global warming, which is the result of fossil fuel use, which is associated with industrialization in Europe and North America.

In the 1990s, the ecologist C.S. "Buzz" Holling brought together an international alliance of scholars to try to understand such complex social-ecological systems. They call themselves the Resilience Alliance and have contributed a great deal to our ability to develop appropriate response and management strategies that will promote both ecological resilience and human well-being. There are other, similar networks, including the International Society for Ecology and Health (EcoHealth for short), the Network for Ecosystem Sustainability and Health (NESH), and the whimsically named Dirk Gently Gang.

These networks are working toward developing a new kind of science capable of asking, and perhaps answering, questions too big to be contained in the laboratory: How can a convivial human existence on the earth be created and prolonged? When that existence ends, what grand, multilayered novel do we wish to tell of our time here on the earth? Will it be a tragedy? A comedy (in the Shakespearean sense of having a happy ending)? Or merely a tawdry television melodrama?

Although I am not an alarmist with apocalyptic visions of the Black Death wiping out modern civilization, I do know that the stories that move national policies today—tales of competitiveness and economic efficiency, economies of scale and unfettered trade—are also tales of sloppy biological thinking. Current national and international policies in the 1990s will most assuredly open the doors for more interesting, more devastating, and more widespread epidemics of disease. The word "plague," according to our best prognostications, shall remain an essential ingredient for intelligent discourse for many centuries to come.

The stories we choose, and the responses to disease, are not scientific choices. They are moral animals, with scientific organs and possibly tragic consequences. If we continue to act fast and loose with our technology and drugs, we may be left without a technology to save us and with the words of Albert Camus ringing in our ears:

> None the less, he knew that the tale he had to tell could not be one of final victory. It could only be the record of what had had to be done, and what assuredly would have to be done again in the never ending fight against terror and its relentless onslaughts, despite their personal afflictions, by all who, while unable to be saints but refusing to bow down to pestilences, strive their utmost to be healers.
>
> ALBERT CAMUS, *The Plague*

(4)

THE WORLD LOOKING AT ITSELF

*F*LEAS ARE not the only arthropods to have teamed up with small rodents with the sole purpose, it seems, of annoying people; nor is the plague the only disease to have taken advantage of this multispecies collaboration to make the leap from other animals to people. Lyme disease has few of the terrifying overtones of the plague, and not a few people have confused the issue by thinking Lyme referred to a fruit and not to a town in Connecticut. But this so-called emerging zoonosis, and the ticks associated with it, have much to teach us about what Douglas Adams called life, the universe, and everything.

Many of us who recall pictures in grade school textbooks, or who have gazed dizzily through university microscopes, tend to think of bacteria as tiny spherical or hot-dog-shaped creatures that multiply into grape-like clusters or strings of wieners. They multiply fast, more orgiastically multiplicative than the most virile polygamous rabbit you can imagine. One of my friends, a food microbiologist, has described how one clan of bacteria, *Clostridium perfringens,* can double its population every eight to ten minutes, producing over a million offspring in four hours, and, barring food, water, and temperature constraints, could multiply to fill the entire planet in about forty-eight hours. The god who created bacteria was clearly thumbing his or her nose at the god created by world religions.

Many people think of these little beings as hanging out in bad places, such as slums, poor countries, unbrushed mouth cavities, and insufficiently sprayed kitchen counters. Bacteria are in the air, on your curtains, on the chair, on your food, on your dog, in your underwear. My goodness, how do we even stay alive? Not content with creating colonial blobs at the back of the refrigerator, bacteria not only use animals, people, and hamburgers as public transit vehicles, but some have even developed their own wheels, so to speak.

According to the microbial ecologist Lynn Margulis, very early in evolution some techno-wizards of the bacterial world developed whip-like tails that are spun around by little proton motors. The motors are propelled by changes of electrical charge. The general term for these motorized tails is "undulopodia." In bacteria (like *Salmonella*) and sperm cells (which are probably just bacteria adapted to warm, moist, and pleasurable places), these are called flagella. In your nostrils and trachea, the smaller, waving, hair-like things that push mucus and dead bacterial bodies up the tubes and into the great recycling heap of the biological world are called cilia.

These are all quite interesting. More interesting for our story, however, are those in which the motors were internalized, which took bacteria from having motorbikes to being little sports cars. When the whip-like twisting filaments became internalized, these bacteria, now called spirochetes, were transformed into the fastest-moving dudes of the microcosm. These fast movers took off to newer, warmer, greener pastures, leaving the old, immobile stick-in-the-muds to survive or die at the whims of local conditions.

Margulis hypothesizes that when spirochetes joined the human Borg colony, they became the cells that make up our brains and nervous systems and the rods and cones of our eyes. This development means that when we look through a microscope at spirochetes, we are nothing more or less than bacteria looking at bacteria, trying to understand ourselves. Reading this statement, I start to feel a little not-myself, dizzy, and a little, if you please, used. But I suppose human beings don't have much of a leg to stand on when they complain to the cosmic court about feeling used.

Although many of these spirochetes are of interest only to those poor folks like myself who are dumbstruck at the wonderfulness of the world, or to dentists with microscopes spelunking in your mouth, a few are downright bothersome. The one that causes syphilis (*Treponema pallidum*), the dark twin of sperm cells, has been a perennial troublemaker, although my wife once worked in a nursing home where an old lady with terminal syphilis appeared to go into a state of near euphoria whenever she was bathed, which would seem to be a better way to die than some others I can think of. I hasten to add that neurosyphilis is not always so benign, and the road to get there can be quite painful, so I can't recommend it as a general solution to the ailments of our mortality.

Two other spirochetes—*Borrelia burgdorferi*, which gives us Lyme disease, and the leptospires, which give us the most common zoonotic disease in the world (not surprisingly called leptospirosis)—are of special interest to zoonotic-disease people. Because they require ticks to complete their life cycle, I'll deal with the *Borrelia* here. I'll come back to the leptospires in a later chapter.

In the mid-1970s, a couple of mothers from Old Lyme, Connecticut, began keeping track of what local physicians had diagnosed as juvenile rheumatoid arthritis. It seemed to these mothers strange that this disease, generally considered rare, should be clustered in their village and in the neighboring villages of Lyme and East Haddam. The persistence of these mothers finally paid off when their story was picked up by Allen Steere, a post-doctoral fellow in rheumatology at the Yale University School of Medicine, who had completed training in epidemiology with the Centers for Disease Control and Prevention in Atlanta. The subsequent story unfolded through a combination of good luck and doggedly good normal science, as researchers wrote down histories of patients, took blood samples, caught ticks from epidemic and non-epidemic areas, and cultured and tested for everything they could think of.

Willy Burgdorfer, an internationally recognized expert on tick-borne diseases, was actually looking for something else among the crushed remains of a tick on his microscope slide. He was looking for small organisms called rickettsiae, which cause Rocky Mountain spotted fever, the same organism that Herald Cox, at the same institution, was looking for when he cultivated the cause of Q fever (see discussion of poker players' pneumonia in chapter 14). Instead of rickettsiae, Burgdorfer saw spiral-shaped bacteria.

The spirochetes Burgdorfer saw, in the same general class as those that cause leptospirosis and syphilis, came to be called *Borrelia burgdorferi*. Further testing showed that they were, indeed, the immediate cause of Lyme disease. The medical and scientific community patted itself on the back for discovering what is now thought to be the most common arthropod-borne zoonosis in North America. Nobody likes to talk about the fact that it would not have been discovered if it hadn't been for a few very persistent, annoying mothers and what this means for how science really works. Few talked about the fact that the Europeans—the Swedes, in particular—had known about the target-rash form of the disease since the early part of the twentieth century and had discovered that it responded well to penicillin. Scientists, I suppose, are as self-absorbed and lacking in humility as anyone else.

We can think about this disease in a variety of ways. Most people, like the mothers in Connecticut, think of it as a disease that affects individual people or animals. That it certainly is.

Infection with *Borrelia burgdorferi* (now referred to in scientific papers as borreliosis, thus further airbrushing the moms from this picture) causes problems not just in individual people. It also affects dogs, horses, and several other species of animals. Several days to a month after the initial injection of the organism from an infected tick about the size of a rice grain or a poppy seed, people may develop a target-shaped rash and some flu-like symptoms such as fever and general pain. The disease seems to respond readily to various antibiotics at this stage. If not treated, the spirochetes swim through the blood and get stuck in tiny capillary laneways, where they cause heart problems, arthritis, neurological problems, and musculoskeletal pain.

Studies by Richard Ostfeld and other ecologists demonstrate that the natural life cycle of *Borrelia burgdorferi* involves field mice, deer, and oak trees. Once every three to four years, oak trees put out a very large acorn crop (called masting). These acorns, rich in fats and proteins, attract field mice and deer that feed on them. The mice also love to feed on the pupae of gypsy moths, a natural pre-emptive strike preventing the moths from attacking the oak tree. Adult ticks, usually some variety of *Ixodes*, drop off the deer where they have been feeding and lay some eggs. The eggs hatch and the larvae feed on the mice, from whom they pick up the spirochete *Borrelia burgdorferi*. After a good blood feed, the larval ticks molt into nymphs, which, the following spring, latch on to whatever fast-food outlet happens to wander into their territory: mice, birds, dogs, hikers, and hunters looking for deer. Late in the summer (or, until recent warming trends, the following year, in some colder places like Canada), the nymphs become adults, and another cycle begins.

From a "rare" affliction in the 1970s, Lyme disease has become the most commonly diagnosed tick-borne disease in North America. Americans now see more than twenty thousand cases per year. In Canada, the number of cases has also begun to creep up, although not as dramatically as farther south. Why is this disease spreading, and what, if anything, can be done about it?

Based on a general understanding of the ecology of the disease, a natural history of Lyme disease in North America might go something like this: Early settlers arrived in New England, and, disturbing the natural life cycles of *Borrelia burgdorferi*, mice, trees, deer, and so on, acquired a variety of aches, pains, and diseases, which were the normal accoutrements of being human. They cleared the forest habitat to make way for farms, and the deer populations dwindled, as did the disease and human memory of it. In the 1970s, economic policies based on abstractions created in the ethereal minds of a few academic economists and on the greed of corporate speculators combined with the lure and food needs of big cities to encourage fewer, larger farms (the so-called economies of scale). Thousands of farms were sold or abandoned in New England (and across North America) and often transformed into "country properties."

This economic disaster for farm families was a major success from some other environmental and social perspectives. Sub-urban "country" dwellers, weaned on Bambi and that family of friendly mice the Littles, decided that nature, especially nature full of non-threatening, picturesque species and devoid of serious predators such as wolf packs and hunters in bright orange vests, was a good thing. As a result, forests made a comeback in New England, along with deer and field mice and a lot of people going for walks in the woods.

All this social and ecological change, furthermore, occurred in a social milieu in which no one is allowed to be just plain tired or full of aches and pains. Clinical disease without a diagnosis is now often stigmatized as hypochondria, and a variety of generalized, non-specific ills, ranging from chronic fatigue syndrome to AIDS to generalized environmental allergies, have come to be defined as diseases.

Diagnosis is a big problem for all zoonoses. Few have typically distinctive signs; the target-shaped rash of Lyme disease, which reflects infection with the organisms at the site of the tick bite, only happens in a quarter of the cases. A history of being bitten by a tick is helpful, but since the ticks are so small, most people don't remember that event, momentous as it is in the life of the tick. The laboratory tests can be unreliable; some of them are plagued with false positives (the test is positive, but the disease is not present), while others have false negatives (the test comes up negative even when the spirochete is touring the bloodstream).

TABLE 1

	DISEASE POSITIVE	DISEASE NEGATIVE	TOTAL
TEST POSITIVE	99	909	1,008
TEST NEGATIVE	1	89,991	98,992
TOTAL	100	90,900	100,000

Even the very best tests do badly if the disease is rare. It is worth doing a little technical aside here. Look carefully at Table 1. The sensitivity of a test is the proportion of those who actually *have* the disease who test positive; we ask, if you have the disease, will you test positive? The specificity is the proportion of those who *don't* have the disease who test negative. These characteristics are pretty stable.

They also, often, involve trade-offs. Let me take an extreme case: If I said that all men have prostate cancer (my test being sex classification), then my sensitivity would be 100 percent; that is, every person who has prostate cancer will be correctly classified as having prostate cancer. Unfortunately, I will also have falsely classified a whole lot of healthy men as cancer positive; that is, the test has a very low specificity. If I say that no men have prostate cancer, then every man who does *not* have prostate cancer will be correctly classified (specificity = 100 percent), but my sensitivity will be zero, since no one with the actual disease will be correctly classified.

Looking across the table at predictive values, we discover something different. A positive predictive value asks, if you test positive, how likely are you to have the disease? The answer to this question depends not only on the sensitivity of the test but also on how common it is, its prevalence. Let us suppose (as in table 1) that Lyme disease occurs in one in every thousand people (100 out of every 100,000 people in the table), which, as diseases go, is pretty high (in Canada, salmonellosis occurs in about 25 out of 100,000 people; *E. coli*-related disease occurs in 3 to 5 out of 100,000). Let us say that we have a test that is 99 percent sensitive (it correctly picks up 99 percent of those who actually have the disease, but it misses 1 percent) and 99 percent specific (it correctly classifies 99 percent of those who are disease free, but it also throws 1 percent of the healthy people into the diseased category), which is better than almost any test on the market for any disease. If only one in a thousand people actually has Lyme disease, then less than 10 percent of those who test positive actually have it. If 90 percent of the people in the population have the disease (flip the "positive" and "negative" columns around), then about 90 percent of those who test positive actually have it.

Mull this over. You have the best test in the world and it is usually wrong on test positives; on the other hand, if the test says you don't have the disease, you probably don't. This is why tests for genetic screening in the general population are much more often wrong than right.

Thus, it is important to know how common the disease is in the area before you test. If a disease is more common, then your test will perform better. But how do you know how common the disease is unless you test? This dilemma—that we depend on tests to describe the true state of the world, but we don't know how well the tests are performing unless we know the truth to begin with—is one of the big reasons that our scientific knowledge always increases much more slowly than the events we are studying. Our understanding of a disease depends on comparing many different kinds of tests over time and a good knowledge of the biology of the species involved. If there is a large population of people with undiagnosed ailments, practicing physicians, under pressure to do something, are strongly tempted either to lump them all into the "diseased" category or to dismiss them as hypochondriacs.

There's no quick fix for this kind of problem. Since tests for diseases always perform better where the diseases are more common, progress depends on asking questions related to where the organism and its associated disease are more likely to be found. Are there social and ecological clues that will help us make the tests perform better?

Ostfeld and his colleagues determined that Lyme disease was less likely to occur in more biologically diverse habitats, since the ticks and the bacteria they were carrying were less likely to be able to find suitable hosts on which they could feed in such habitats. Buzz Holling and his colleagues in the Resilience Alliance would say that diverse habitats, which buffer against disease, are resilient, meaning that they have the ability to adapt and change and continually reorganize themselves in the context of a changing world. Members of the EcoHealth network might refer to it as ecosystem health, which means something similar. Whatever term is used to describe this ability to have long, healthy, friendly lives on this planet, we are losing it, not just through loss of biodiversity but also through human-induced climate changes.

So the disease is more likely to be found where the deer are plentiful and the field mice and the ticks can live out their full lives as expeditiously as possible—in warm places with as few species competing for food and housing as possible. Unfortunately, by most accounts, we are creating conditions in a lot of places where Lyme disease is more likely to occur. This development may be good for people who are worried about test performance, but it is bad news for those of us out for a walk in the woods.

Our own research team, led by the veterinary entomologist Nicholas Ogden, studied temperature and microhabitat effects on tick development and linked those effects to projected climate changes. We already knew that Lyme disease had a strong foothold in two southern parks of Canada—Long Point and Point Pelee—in part because those are major transit points for thousands of migrating birds every spring and fall and in part because the temperature, moisture, and general ecological conditions were right. We already knew that those areas had white-tailed deer and field mice, both necessary for the disease to establish itself. We also knew that migrating birds carried ticks (so-called adventitious ticks), which dropped off throughout their migration routes, like passengers getting off airplanes at various destinations.

Because of these adventitious ticks, we occasionally saw cases of Lyme disease scattered throughout Canada, well away from areas considered to be endemic. So far, we had little evidence that the ticks and the disease they carried were being established in local, home-grown cycles. The question we asked was: how important would milder winters and hotter summers be in the northward movement of Lyme disease?

To get the ticks, Ogden and fellow researcher Robbin Lindsay took four male research dogs out into the woods at Long Point, one of the southernmost areas of Canada. Robbin, an intrepid entomologist with the Public Health Agency of Canada's secure laboratory in Winnipeg, who had battled the prairie mosquito swarms, tramped through jungles in Africa, and spelunked in the dank sewers in Windsor, Ontario (where he found overwintering mosquitoes harboring West Nile virus), thought he had seen just about everything. The theory was that the four beagles would attract ticks, which would then be picked off and studied under controlled laboratory and field conditions. Unfortunately (for our study), two of the more dominant dogs took a keen sexual interest in the third dog, who was apparently giving off receptive messages. Nick and Robbin were left dragging an entangled threesome, plus the fourth dog, who seemed to be of the more traditional alpha male Christian Heritage family variety.

In the end, they managed to get enough ticks to run the experiments, although some of the ticks escaped the escape-proof containers we had designed for them. One of our research assistants, Matthew Waltner-Toews (and yes, related), was not surprised. He recounted tales of how, during monitoring of bird populations at Cape Cod, the tiny ticks would manage to slip down undetected inside the socks-over-pants, into the shoes, and back up the legs into dark and moist and unmentionable places. Our field experiments demonstrated that the ticks did very well in most environments, even our most severe ("control") sites, and that temperature seemed to be the major driving force for tick development. In part, what was protecting Canadians and other northerners from diseases like Lyme disease was a cold winter.

From our study (and others) it became clear that warmer weather associated with climate change is already encouraging the ticks and the disease to migrate northward into parts of Canada where they were formerly seen only rarely. If the climate and environment were stable, we could develop public health and management strategies to deal with diseases where they occur endemically. By altering the climate and the environment, we are changing the baseline and encouraging diseases to spread into new areas. In other words, our ability to adapt is being undermined by the way in which we continually change the environment to which we are trying to adapt. Driving cars is connected to global climate change, which is connected to local weather change, which is connected to the spread of disease in landscapes transformed through agricultural and economic policies and urban and peri-urban planning and landscape development activities. The possible strategies to deal with this problem are discussed in the final chapters of the book, since the success of responses to one disease problem is very much connected to how we solve a whole lot of other problems.

(5)

BITING FLIES, KISSING BUGS,

AND SLEEPING SICKNESS

*N*OT ALL arthropods have cast their lots with the rodents. Some of them, the biting flies that carry parasites that cause sleeping sickness and kala-azar among them, have gone upscale on the evolutionary ladder.

One of a family of diseases caused by a genus of slinky, willow-leaf-like blood parasites called trypanosomes, sleeping sickness is one of those African diseases that have perplexed and frightened people for many centuries. The parasites, members of a class of living things called Euglenozoa, are descended from some of the oldest living things with nuclei (eukaryotes). They are thought to be about 300 million years old, which takes us back to the Paleozoic era (roughly 543 to 248 million years ago), a world of swamps, explosions of a brilliant, exuberant diversity of all forms of animal life, and wandering supercontinents, when Africa and South America were still joined at the hip. The era ended catastrophically (as many seem to, sadly reflecting a somewhat ill-tempered Creator), with a breaking up and drifting apart of the continents and, one might suggest, an incontinent flood of species extinctions (90 percent, some suggest). This early birth of the trypanosome species explains why there are different genuses, with different ecologies, but similar ancestries, in South America and Africa. I'll come back to the South American one a bit later.

Tsetse flies, which (in Africa) now transmit the parasites from one tropically warm bloodstream to another, seem to go back about 200 million years, to Mesozoic times (some 248 to 65 million years ago). That era gave us ferns, cycads, ginkgophytes, bennettitaleans, and other unusual plants, as well as conifers and angiosperms (a curious name, with etymological scents of blood vessels [angio] and male reproduction; some with a more prosaic turn of phrase would call them flowering plants, which provide us with pretty well all the foods and many of the drugs we rely on), but also Jurassic Park and the oil deposits of the North Sea. Sadly, it also ended with a mass extinction, which took down not only the dinosaurs but also the ammonites, who I once fondly dreamed might have been the forebears to Mennonites, who begat me. Alas, not so. According to some sources, these marine mollusks succumbed on the Maastrichtian stage in, one would imagine, a dramatic fashion. The stage is named after the site in the Netherlands where chalk rocks typical of this era are found and where the Treaty on European Union was staged and signed in 1992, although it would be stretching credibility to argue for some sort of evolutionary connection here.

So both the parasites and the flies are survivors. We humans are newcomers on the scene, a mere five million or so years ago, and probably just picked up the parasite when we started farming and herding cattle in risky landscapes. For thousands of years, people and parasites lived in a kind of loose truce, people tending to avoid tsetse fly habitats and clearing brush from around their houses. Our written records of the flies (probably) go back to the Jewish prophet Isaiah of the early to mid-700s BC, who wrote: "In that day, the Lord will whistle for flies from the distant streams of Egypt... They will come and settle in the steep ravines and in the crevices in the rocks, on all the thorn bushes and at all the water holes" (Is. 7:18–19, New International Version). The image of this Old Testament god whistling for flies reconfirms the adage of some biologists that the creator seemed inordinately fond of insects.

The Muslim historian Ibn Khaldoun in 1406 reported not just on the annoying flies but also on the disease itself. There were reports from Mali that a king suffered two years of profound sleep on the throne (did no one notice?) before he finally died of the disease. Khaldoun apparently picked up this information from traders crossing the Sahara. Certain tribes in western Africa apparently had about fifty names for the disease, which, if one might draw a parallel to the many names for "snow" northerners are said to have, or names for "sand" among desert dwellers, indicates either very close familiarity with the disease or a culture where people have much idle time on their hands. Our scientific knowledge of the parasite increased rapidly in the nineteenth and early twentieth centuries, when it began to interfere with the slave trade and hindered European trashing of Africa.

As one might imagine, the trypanosome ancestors probably evolved, much as people have, from free-living swimmers to parasites of non-human animals (about five million years ago). Some subspecies only affect wildlife and domestic cattle. The Zulus named the animal disease "nagana," meaning "a state of depressed spirits," which pretty well sums it up. Two members of the species *Trypanosoma brucei*, however, can be shared between other animals and people. *T. brucei gambiense* generally lives in western Africa, and the disease it causes unfolds slowly and inexorably, a bit, perhaps, like nagana. This species of the parasite is fully adapted to living in and spreading between people, the city cousin that has no interest in returning to the wild. Other species only infect animals, which are of interest to veterinarians and as historical artifacts but not as zoonoses. For those interested in genealogy, the earliest trypanosomes were probably adapted to wildlife, in which many of them, to this day, seem to cause few problems. The zoonotic form (*T. brucei rhodesiense*) emerged later, probably in the Ionian (also known as the Middle Pleistocene) epoch, tens to hundreds of thousands of years ago. Still later (say, ten thousand years ago), the human-adapted form, *T. brucei gambiense*, emerged.

The interesting member of this family of blood parasites, from the point of view of emergence of disease, ecology, and our stumbling attempts to define a convivial niche for ourselves on the planet, is *T. brucei rhodesiense*. This one lives mostly in eastern and central Africa and causes acute fever, aches and pains, and general miserableness. The body's immune system attacks the parasites, but these little guerrillas have complicated, multi- and mini-circles of DNA, including one thousand genes (which also mutate, creating more) coding for different surface coats. Just when the body thinks it has defeated them, they come back in different uniforms, and the battle starts again; the immune system is at first very active and later exhausted. Toward the end, the parasites slink their way across the blood-brain barrier into the king's castle and start messing with people's minds.

Classically, human sleeping sickness starts with a flu-like illness and proceeds through disrupted sleep patterns to the final sleep of an irreversible coma—hence the name—but psychoses and aggression are not unheard of, and patients have inadvertently ended up in prisons and mental hospitals. The World Health Organization estimates that there are upward of 300,000 cases in people a year. In the region in eastern Uganda, which I visited as part of a research team in 2001, about twelve thousand people have died since 1986.

This "Rhodesian" sleeping sickness can be carried around by a lot of different animals, including cattle, where it may stay cryptic or cause nagana. These trypanosomes are carried from animal to animal and to people by tsetse flies, which, like many sensible animals in the tropics, prefer to live in shady places, especially near waterways. The female fly, perhaps having been schooled by thrifty Scottish Presbyterians, breeds once and then, with almost obsessive thrift, saves the sperm and uses it as she needs it. I have no information about what must surely be the onanistic, lonely habits of the males. The female fly lays an egg every nine days in moist, loose ground, and the new flies emerge about three weeks later. This reproductive frugality flies in the face of the "logic" of reckless child production systems, which have allowed humanity to fill and dominate the earth but are now threatening the whole wonderful biospheric experiment. The flies have been around for a lot longer than us, and we might reconsider our strategies.

Context, of course, is everything.

On May 28, 2000, the day before my fifty-second birthday, I was sitting on the deck at the home of Catherine Kenyatta, gregarious, gracious, cheerful granddaughter of Jomo Kenyatta, founder of modern Kenya, and her husband, Sean. We were in Mbale, eastern Uganda. A motley crew of researchers from Kenya, Canada, Zambia, England, Scotland, and Uganda, we were there to work with the Ugandans to try to understand, and control, the re-emergence of sleeping sickness in eastern Africa.

The view from where I nursed my beer was across the darkening shadow of the town to the foothills of Mount Elgon. I would say it was evening, but readers in temperate zones might confuse this with the slow draining of color that occurs at dusk. There, I could already sense the black pixels gathering under leaves, in the shadows of huts and palms. When they reached some critical point, the whole landscape would suddenly cascade into darkness. I wondered if this difference in the experience of diurnal change might explain the faith among many temperate zone scientists in gradually changing ecosystems (global warming degree by degree, increments of pollution, slowly rising epidemics) and blinding them to critical points, collapses, and sudden changes, which characterize pretty well all the world's ecosystems and may give us clues as to how to prevent emergent epidemics.

From a distance, the nearest hill rose up in red-gray-black cliffs to a plateau, waterfalls spraying down crevices, shaggy green tatters like carpets stuck precariously to the cliff faces. But views from a distance should not be confused with "broader views" and may be misleading; sometimes distance gives not perspective but fuzzy thinking.

That afternoon, veterinary epidemiologist John McDermott, geographer Barry Smit, and I had clambered up one of those steep slopes. Up close, every fold and wrinkle of the hillside was inhabited by villages and farms, kids, goats, men and women washing carrots in a stream. The green patches on the cliff faces were farmers' fields. Barry, a Kiwi-cum-Canadian, aspiring sheep farmer, co-author of reports from the Intergovernmental Panel on Climate Change, does not suffer fools or idle activities gladly. Unlike me, he dislikes activities without a clear purpose. He therefore gave our walk a purpose, identifying an end (some caves high up on the slopes), and things to learn on the way (asking our guides all about the crops being grown).

I was at first annoyed at this intrusion into my non-doing, thoughtless, mind-clearing activity. I was soon captivated, however, as Barry asked again and again: What is this? Why are they growing that? In those scant, thin soils clinging to the rocks, farmers were growing: Irish potatoes (three kinds); yams (four kinds); sweet potatoes; cabbage; carrots; cassava; bananas (one kind for eating; another kind where the fruit was inedible but the sap from the stem was used for treating measles); plants to treat malaria and gonorrhea; peas; beans; pumpkins; leguminous trees; napier grass for erosion control, cattle feed, and mulching; eucalyptus for fuel and soil control; onions; coffee; and at least two kinds of trees near houses to serve as lightning rods. I was in awe of this managed complexity and the possibility for hope for our species that this human-modified landscape embodied.

Buzz Holling and his Resilience Alliance have described the developmental path of many such linked social-ecological systems as moving through natural phases of growth, conservation, creative destruction, and reorganization. Such systems, the systems we live in and are part of, can recover from destruction such as fires and disease outbreaks if that destruction is localized, embedded in a larger, resilient system that can, through a variety of networks and feedback loops, provide nutrients, genetic material, and energy for renewal. The larger system "learns" from the smaller outbreaks and in turn uses this learning to respond to other local outbreaks and fires elsewhere in the larger system. This learning is embodied not just in biological and genetic diversity but also in social and cultural diversity and in the links and communications that exist among these diverse elements. This idea of many small catastrophes embedded in a larger resilient set of systems is sometimes referred to as a shifting steady-state mosaic. Individuals die and families suffer, but the biosphere continues to make a home for our descendants. In a sense, the nature of which we are a part is a kind of flexible, responsive, diverse welfare state.

For farmers in the tropics, maintaining various diverse crops means that they can more easily adapt to changing market, social, and climate conditions around them. If some parts of the system crash (prices of certain crops, the crops themselves), there is enough redundancy of function in their collective agroecosystems that some of them will be okay most of the time, they can take care of each other, and, collectively, they can ride out the crash, learn from it, and keep going. It is also quite certain that a diverse ecosystem provides some protection against disease epidemics; if a variety of crops serving similar functions (providing food, healing, material for building) are grown, and a variety of animals, including those that eat insects, inhabit that agro-ecosystem, then bacteria, viruses, and parasites don't have the equivalent of one of those all-you-can-eat "trough" restaurants that are so beloved by many Americans and that monocultures freely provide.

Although diversity protects against the spread of epidemics and pandemics, however, it can, in some circumstances (when people invade new territories, for instance), foster the emergence of new troublemaking microbes, as the story of avian influenza demonstrates. The trick is to find ways to foster diversity-related resilience without promoting diversity-related disease. It is possible, but it will require us to go well beyond the ecologically simplistic thinking embedded in the either-or mindsets of "progressive, scientific economics of scale" versus "old-fashioned, subsistence poverty."

When we reached the end of our walk, up near the ridge of the mountain, we stepped into a cool, dank cave, once used by rebels during the time of Idi Amin. For a moment we stood there—John, Barry, the two guides, and I—bent over in the low dusk of the cave. Then, Barry's clear tenor voice echoed around us, singing the haunting Righteous Brothers song "Unchained Melody." We stood in silence, as if this were some kind of religious ritual, which, I supposed later, it was. Then we walked back down the mountain.

That night, I lay on my back and pondered the options available to the Ugandans—available to *us*, if I am to count myself as a fellow human being—for dealing with zoonotic sleeping sickness. Smit, myself, and the others were here because McDermott had put together an international research team to answer the question: "Links between sleeping sickness and natural resource endowments and use: what can communities do?" What indeed? I thought.

We could wait until people were sick and then treat them. But finding sick people early and treating them aggressively with toxic drugs is not a program with a high chance of success in central and eastern Africa. For one thing, this is not the plague, and the drug of choice is not some benign antibiotic. Some suggested that the treatment for sleeping sickness felt like having an infusion of red-hot chili peppers. Médecins sans Frontières had enough trouble getting pharmaceutical companies to produce and provide the drugs and then putting them to use, against the much simpler problem of human-adapted *gambiense* sleeping sickness.

We could try to get rid of all the animals that are carrying the parasite. This had been tried before, both by people (as in game destruction) and by that unpredictable god who rules the earth. In 1896, an epidemic of rinderpest, caused by a virus that is probably the ancestor of measles in people and distemper in dogs, swept through southern and eastern Africa, killing millions of cattle and big game. The parasites, in a small-is-beautiful move that presaged the economic philosophy of E.F. Schumacher, survived in the small, numerous, adaptable bushpigs and bushbucks, as well as spending more time among people.

We could spray massive amounts of pesticides to kill the flies or cut down all the shady places where the flies like to breed, but those strategies had already been tried. In the 1950s, before there were subjects like biology in school, both knapsack sprayers and airplanes were used. And clearing all the brush along streams is also a non-starter. Poor communities who live near rivers and depend on cattle and wildlife for food are not usually keen on destroying the places where they live in order to get rid of a disease.

The big outbreaks of sleeping sickness in the twentieth century happened during periods of social upheaval—the early and late years of Idi Amin's terrible reign, for instance. In these times there was breakdown of health and agricultural infrastructure, along with widespread violence. During the fighting, people fled their homes; after the fighting, they returned, bringing with them cattle from southern, infected territories. When raiders from Sudan in the north rustled those cattle away, the people brought in more infected cattle.

Now, in the post-Amin years, Eric Fèvre, Lea Berrang Ford, and other members of our research team found that new areas were becoming infected as cattle were moved into them from the south. After entering a new area, the parasites and tsetse flies spread out along waterways and other fly-friendly habitats. Our big concern was that the *rhodesiense* parasite was moving into territory normally inhabited by the human-adapted *gambiense*, with complicated consequences for diagnoses and control. Could the epidemic be stopped? The diversity of the farms we had seen on the hillside reflected a newfound optimism among Ugandans, which was also expressed in a vibrant local democracy. This optimism, coupled with civic engagement, offered some hope for finally coming to terms with the old parasite.

Still, the disease presented itself as what is sometimes called a "smoldering" epidemic: the infection spread inexorably through the countryside, but clinical cases were always at a level low enough to stay just under the radar. On the one hand, a low number of cases seemed to be a good thing. On the other hand, for people resettling land and struggling to get past decades of war and destruction, a few cases here and there hardly provided motivation to mount major control programs. The old top-down approaches of technocrats telling locals what to do didn't have much support; the people at the top didn't have the money to sustain such a program, and the people on the ground had other things on their minds and had had enough of others telling them what to do.

The day after our trek up the mountain, we piled into our vehicles and headed out past open fields north toward Soroti, catching glimpses of Lake Kyoga, and over rutted, dusty roads where weather-beaten villagers huddled next to burlap sacks of charcoal, to a group of mud and thatch huts gathered in the shade of a grove of trees. This was to be our medical research post for the day. We set up tables with centrifuges and blood collection tubes. Some of us interviewed farmers under a tree. Men from the village, joined by researchers, wrestled with the cows, checking ears and testicles for ticks (lots of them), taking tubes of blood from the jugular and sucking up a tiny bit from the ear into a glass capillary tube.

Women, men, children lined up under the trees, forming a winding line around the village, all to be questioned, examined by a nurse or doctor, and have blood taken. Cattle milled about in the shade of various trees in the vicinity. Children cried, cattle in heat clambered on to each other and tried to breed. One young cow chased a dog around and around, trying with its nose and tongue to determine the nature of this shy creature. Children stood in a circle around me as I did a second reading on hemoglobin color tests for the medical technologist. They were most fascinated when she injected blood from cows, suspected of being infected, into mice, where it could be kept alive for later molecular studies. The mice, held by the loose skin on their necks, looked open-mouthed with surprise.

Near lunch, in the heat of the day, I went out with three other fellows to hang traps for tsetse flies. We wandered down a sun-beaten path to the swampy area near the river, one of the spidery fingers of water draining into Lake Kyoga. The soft ground was crisscrossed with deep ruts, paths from people and animals looking for water. I wished I had my Tilley hat, and I carried the traps over my head for protection from the blistering sun. The traps are like tents, with white mesh at the peak and blue and black cloth at the base, since tsetse flies are attracted to black and dark shades of blue. Thus, there was some poignancy is seeing schoolkids wearing blue and black shorts and tops clearly made from fly-attracting traps, which underlined the urgency of engaging local populations in the enterprise, combining education with action.

When the flies reach the colored lower part of the trap, they fly up toward the light, through small holes, and into the top part, where they are trapped. We hung the traps from trees in shady areas, often near water. I didn't pay much attention to the first water hole we came to, thinking it to be a dugout for cattle.

At the second or third dugout we visited, there were several women, bent over, letting the brown liquid burble into their bright canary-yellow jerry cans. I asked about the coffee-latte-colored water in the hole. Was this for drinking?

"Yes," said the ten-year-old kid who was showing us around.

"Without boiling?"

He demonstrated how to clear away the flotsam and insects at the surface, scoop it into your hand, and drink it. "But not for you," he grinned. "You will get sick."

The two other men with us, who were from outside the area, also said they would be sick if they drank that water. I thought of the people in Walkerton, Ontario, where thousands had been sickened in May 2000 by drinking "clear" tap water; several died. Pausing beside a termite mound six feet or more high, the boy grinned at me as he dug away with a stick, pointing out the big, angry termite guards that came out to challenge his intrusions. When fried, he assured me, they were excellent with sesame paste.

This is why I am here, I mused. A sense not so much of home, or necessarily of saving the world (although we would all like to do that, I suppose), but of camaraderie, of being on an incredible journey together, of being part of something wonderful, bigger than all of us, of trying to make a not-too-uncomfortable place for ourselves in the midst of the messy, complex, amazing world we live in. Of promoting health, defined by the late, great microbiologist René Dubos as "modus vivendi enabling imperfect [people] to achieve a rewarding and not too painful existence while they cope with an imperfect world."

Returning from hanging the traps, we found that the others had already eaten lunch. I stood under a tree, wiping the sweat from my forehead, and drank a Coke. I recalled the Coca-Cola sign at the equator, when we had driven over from Kenya the previous week. I had thought then, and I thought now, that one of my motivations for being here was to provide a counterweight, to help people find an alternative story, to that of the ubiquitous Coca-Cola-type McEmpires. But out there in the sun, damn, was I thirsty.

On the evening of May 29, 2000, at the Sunrise Restaurant in Mbale, I looked around the table at our sunburned, disheveled group and reflected once more on the web of narratives and motives that had drawn us there. We looked over the menu, and someone asked what a White Russian was. I did not, then, recount my entire family history, the revolution, the civil war, the fleeing of wealthy farmers from Stalin's bureaucratic utopia, that ultimate in top-down scientific technocratic solutions. But I did think then that my own personal story was part of this larger story, that every researcher is part of what he or she does research on, that sustainable health and development are all about finding a common journey and a Chaucerian story we can tell each other on the way. What passed my lips was something like, "Did you know that my parents fled from the Soviet Union in 1926? And now here I am in Uganda, on my birthday."

The British epidemiologist Paul Coleman's response to this statement was to order a round of White Russians, with the rule that I would have to finish the drinks of all those who didn't. As a benediction, somewhat inebriated, fresh from a day in the field and beers at Catherine and Sean's, emotional (I hesitate to call it maudlin, but perhaps it was), scrounging through my topsy-turvy mind for a succinct summing-up of this out-of-the-lab-

and-into-the-world science, my mental and physical transports from Canada to Mbale, I could think of no better response to the complex history of sleeping sickness, and our challenge to come to some convivial, ecologically negotiated truce with it, than to recite the poem "Wild Geese," by Mary Oliver, a wonderful evocation of wild geese flying overhead and their "harsh and exciting" message to us that we are all part of the same family.

TRYPANOSOMES IN THE Western Hemisphere took a somewhat different path to finding a home. Chagas disease, named after Carlos Chagas, one of the world's great biomedical investigators, is a kind of distant cousin to African sleeping sickness. It is sometimes called American sleeping sickness, but that is a misnomer, since the disease it causes is nothing like African sleeping sickness. Technically, one could simply call it American trypanosomiasis. As you can imagine, after a few hundred million years of separation, the family resemblance has been somewhat diluted. Unlike its African cousins, this trypanosome does not cross the blood-brain barrier, so the disease has none of the manifestations associated with infection of the brain. Many people get infected, but not many become ill. In those who do succumb, the heart grows large and flabby, and it can't effectively pump blood anymore. In another form of the disease, the intestines get large and flabby and food pools in the gut. In either case, the victim dies, slowly, painfully, over many years.

One Brazilian researcher, the late Philip Davis Marsden, described the disease as "retribution for colonizing the New World." From Mexico south to Chile and Argentina, some 16 million people are thought to be infected and 75 million at risk. Evidence from dried-out human mummies suggests that the parasite was already cycling among animals and bugs in southern Peru and northern Chile nine thousand years ago, waiting for more humans to come intruding. They did.

For affected individuals, American trypanosomiasis can be described as a disease caused by *Trypanosoma cruzi,* a single-celled blood parasite with an undulating membrane and a tail, not much different in appearance from the other trypanosomes. Swimming through the bloodstream like delicate tropical fish, the parasites nose their way into various body cells, where they lose their tails and, like baby boomers in suburbia, wreak their damage locally. Actual clinical disease associated with these parasites, though not common, may be acute or chronic and involve a wide range of organs, from the heart to the brain to the intestines. It is an important cause of sudden death from cardiomyopathy (pathology of the heart muscles) throughout Latin America and is associated with a chronic ballooning of the intestines that is called megacolon.

From a medical-ecological point of view, there are various cycles of transmission, some restricted to non-human mammals (over a hundred species infected), some crossing into human populations, and some passing from person to person. The traditional means of transport for the trypanosomes is through what have been called "kissing bugs" of the triatomine family. These blood-feeding insects might be tens of millions of years old, but they have adapted well to human invasion of their territories. At night, they quietly emerge from the cracks and crevices where they live and "kiss" people, soundlessly, painlessly, looking for a blood meal, at the corners of their victims' eyes or in small wounds or scratches. The bugs' eyes are bigger than their stomachs, as my mother would have said, and they have to urinate a lot just to keep sucking in the blood. These bugs, not being hygienically fastidious, defecate where they eat. The parasite lives in the triatomid's feces. Rubbing their eyes when they feel the tickle of the bug, people also rub the parasite into their blood. More than fifty species of triatomines can carry the parasite.

From a broader cultural point of view, this is a disease of global politics and power struggles between empires, from the

Europeans and Incas several hundred years ago to the United States and Latin America today. Triatomine bugs originally lived (happily?) in free-living forest mammals in South and Central America. With deforestation, some bugs that were originally sylvatic ("wild," as in Sylvester the cartoon cat) seem to have adapted to more open types of vegetation and have also developed a penchant for certain kinds of human dwellings, thus increasing the frequency of transmission of *T. cruzi* to humans.

These types of poorly constructed (for people, not bugs) dwellings, frequently found crowded into shantytowns, did not occur by mere chance. During the height of the cold war, the United States and the former Soviet Union fought their battles in many poor countries. While the Soviets were subjugating parts of Europe, in Latin America, the U.S. overthrew democratic governments and fought pitched and dirty battles against popular uprisings. These wars drove many people from the countryside to slums around major cities. In recent years, the move from the countryside to the city has been accelerated by neoliberal economic policies, which have tended to favor large, wealthy landowners and to drive peasants into forest areas (and the *T. cruzi* sylvatic cycles) or into the slums (and the *T. cruzi* urban cycles). The slums that have resulted from this combination of military and economic battles are an ideal breeding ground for the triatomid bugs that carry the parasites.

Now, in a new twist on the retribution theme and another warning of how small organisms can adapt more quickly to cultural change than the people who initiated the changes, the parasites recently discovered a new superhighway created by people: blood-bank systems in Latin America in the 1980s were infested with the parasites at rates from 6 percent (Buenos Aires) to 63 percent (Santa Cruz, Bolivia). These blood banks are likely to provide a pathway for the disease to spread from the poor to the wealthy. If they had the brains to anticipate, the parasites would no doubt look forward to a globalized blood supply.

Going to an even larger picture, it seems that changes in climate may have already begun to increase the distribution of one of the insect vectors of Chagas, *T. nigromaculata,* which has been found for the first time at altitudes above 2,600 feet in Venezuela. Infected vectors were first found at 2,600 feet in 1939, but an uninfected colony was found more recently in a modern dwelling at an altitude of more than 3,600 feet in the Venezuelan Andes. So fossil fuel use, which contributes to global warming, can also be considered a cause of the spread of Chagas disease.

In some ways, if the conundrums of diseases such as these can be solved, there is hope that many other difficult global problems can be resolved. Indeed, we may *need* to resolve just about everything in order to solve anything in particular. This is both a good thing and a bad thing. It means that the solutions to disease and food and energy and community may all be part of the same, much larger, more complex solution. If only we can find them.

THE PARASITES THAT cause American and African sleeping sickness are not the only troublemakers in this family of parasites.

From the mid-1980s to the mid-1990s, a couple of hundred thousand people in the southern Sudanese state of Western Upper Nile (also called Unity State by the government in Khartoum) died of what was described as an "AIDS-like" disease. The disease, kala-azar, or visceral leishmaniasis, was being carried by sand flies in acacia forests along flooded rivers. Investigators think soldiers took the infection into an area that had been reforested after destructive floods in the 1960s.

The leishmania are one-celled parasites from the same family as the trypanosomes and thus go back hundreds of millions of years. According to one (well-grounded) story, at least one of the major forms of the parasite has its ancestral home in what is now southern Sudan and spread out with early human migrations into the wider world of central Asia and southern Europe. It was probably living in our faithful hangers-on, domestic dogs.

In the early nineteenth century, there may have been a second African exodus, some parasite-infected animals hitchhiking on the slave trade boats to head east across the Red Sea and into India. A British army physician, William Leishman, discovered the parasite associated with Dum-Dum fever at a military camp at Dum-Dum, outside Calcutta (and where the airport is today). Later, as the creation of tea plantations allowed the disease to spread into Assam State, it was called British government disease. But other forms of the parasite emerged elsewhere. In eighteenth-century Turkey, it was called Aleppo boil. Among the Incas, it (or something like it) was called valley sickness and, paradoxically, Andean sickness. There is evidence that the disease was present in the Americas as far back as the first century AD.

Unlike true (African) sleeping sickness, which is found only in Africa, and Chagas disease, which occurs in the Western Hemisphere, leishmaniasis is a global citizen. Leishmaniasis is one of the world's top ten most important infectious diseases (along with both African and American trypanosomiasis). The World Health Organization's Tropical Disease Research Programme reports that leishmaniasis occurs in eighty-eight countries, including sixteen European nations. There are probably more than a million people infected every year. WHO estimates that almost sixty thousand people die from it every year and that it costs the world more than two million disability-adjusted life years annually.

Up until World War II and the introduction of DDT, serious infections in children were common in Mediterranean Europe. The drop in numbers of people affected was attributed (why not?) to the use of pesticides, but the infection remained in dogs, which means the parasite was still around and reproducing. More likely, the disease in kids disappeared because of better nutrition and improved immunity, the same things that staved off a lot of other diseases (without necessarily stopping infection). HIV, which allows latent infections to become active for many diseases, has helped give leishmaniasis, like tuberculosis, a new lease on life.

These little blood parasites live quite happily, not causing any major problems, in a variety of marsupials, two- and three-toed sloths, armadillos, and forest rodents (in Central and South America), rock hyraxes and African grass rats (in Africa), fat sand rats (in Saudi Arabia), and great gerbils (in Russia, Mongolia, and central Asia). In many countries, domestic dogs carry it, but they get sick enough to suggest that they aren't the natural host. In fact, in 2000, foxhounds in eighteen U.S. states and two Canadian provinces were sick with leishmaniasis, but that strain appeared to be transferred only between dogs directly, and no human cases were reported. In some parts of India and Africa, there appears to be one form that is adapted just to people, but that could be because we haven't looked at the right animal host yet.

Usually—the epidemic in foxhounds notwithstanding—blood-sucking sand flies (of which there are about seventy important dis-ease-transmitting species) pick up the parasites from one animal and carry them to another. People often get the parasite, via the sand flies, from dogs, after the dogs get it from nosing around in the woods. The types of sand flies and the habitats they prefer vary from place to place. They seem to prefer dry areas in the Old World and tropical forests and savannas in the New. In some areas, they prefer large cities with slums and lots of poor people.

A couple of weeks after the female sand fly lays her five or six dozen eggs, they hatch, and the larvae nose around to feed on any kind of organic stuff they can find. They pupate and emerge as adults in darkness, just before the birds' morning song. Indeed, the wiggling larvae may just be the reason why the birds are sing-ing. Male flies encourage females to mate by flapping their wings and giving off odors (what else is new?); both feed on sugary secretions of plants, but only the females suck blood. When not breeding or sucking on things, the flies rest in cool, shady, humid places. If the females suck blood from an infected animal, they get infected.

In sand flies, the parasites are slinky things, each with a flagellum (tail), which allows them to move around and hang on to the fly's gut cells. The parasites need to hang on tightly until about the third day after a blood meal, which is when the fly defecates. Once the fly has had a good dump, the parasites let go, relax, and multiply as fast as they can. They reproduce by dividing down the middle, which seems considerably less pleasurable, but more efficient, than some other means. The newly "born" parasites then swim around anxiously waiting for the fly to take another meal; when that happens, they are off to the big blood meal in the sky: a mammal.

In animals, including people, the parasite invades white blood cells of the immune system, where it loses its tail, rounds itself into a ball and multiplies. Once in an animal, it can do a variety of things, depending on the immune state of the animal, the particular species of *Leishmania,* and a lot of things that aren't yet very well understood. Much of the time, it appears that nothing particularly bad happens.

In other cases, very bad things indeed happen. Sometimes, if the parasite stays on the skin, it causes a reddish, insect-bite-like sore, which can expand into an open, wet sore called an Oriental sore, which looks a bit like a volcano. In some people, especially with one species of parasite in Brazil, the mucous membranes of the mouth or nose may be completely eaten away, sometimes years after the initial invasion. This condition is called espundia. The worst form of the disease is visceral leishmaniasis, in which the little stinkers invade the spleen and liver and cause a wasting-away-until-death-do-us-part scenario.

How do we begin to get a handle on these complicated parasitic diseases? There are the old diagnosis-treatment-vaccination tricks, of course. They are always handy, but they depend on good diagnostic laboratories, vaccines, and drugs—in other words, on money and trained people. These are in short supply in those parts of the world where these parasitic diseases are most common.

In those places where dogs are a major source of the parasites for flies and people, they may offer some opportunities for control. In the late 1980s, one of my graduate students went to investigate an epidemic of leishmaniasis in a town in Central America. She wanted to explore the role of dogs. When she arrived, she found that local authorities had already killed all the dogs, and new ones were being brought in. The Chinese apparently were effective in getting rid of the disease in some places by getting rid of dogs. Dogs, however, are not just carriers of disease or even just human companions. In some countries, they are food. And, as we discovered in our work in Nepal (chapter 16), they may have other jobs, for example as night guards and community police. Even removing rodents or rodent habitats may pose unexpected problems, as discussed in chapter 3.

How, then, can these diseases be prevented? The answers go beyond the community engagement and setting of fly traps that might have a chance for controlling sleeping sickness in Uganda. The biomedical approach would include treating sick people, spraying for bugs, testing people at risk, and screening blood supplies. This might help control the disease; it would also bring large benefits to certain chemical and technical industries in wealthy countries. But any sustainable health program to prevent these diseases would surely quickly become a social activist program. An ecosystemic and socially holistic approach to health will not, contrary to expectations, always create win-win situations. We still have to make moral choices.

Any programs to prevent these diseases caused by blood parasites must include a political agenda to create more egalitarian societies and a more just global distribution of wealth. With better nutrition, fewer people get sick, even if they are infected. With better-built houses, biting flies and bugs can be more easily be kept outside. If people do get sick, good medical care can stop the cycle of reinfection more quickly. It is just such a combination of medical and socio-political programs that seems to be bringing down the incidence of Chagas disease in the southern cone countries (Argentina, Bolivia, Brazil, Chile, Paraguay, and Uruguay).

It remains to be seen whether similar programs can be mounted for leishmaniasis and sleeping sickness, which have a more complex ecology. Given the general ecology of these diseases, we are unlikely ever to be rid of them completely, and the need for supportive medical programs to deal with inevitable tragedies in an overcrowded world is not going to disappear. We are left with a need for both ecological awareness and global solidarity.

Of Singing and Flight

. . .

DISEASES PEOPLE GET *from*

ANIMALS, INVOLVING BIRDS,

WITH *or* **WITHOUT ARTHROPODS**

. . .

(6)

WESTERN EQUINE ENCEPHALITIS,

TELEVISION, AND AIR CONDITIONING

*T*HE DECLARATION of victory over infectious diseases in the 1970s, from the helm of the smallpox eradication aircraft carrier, was premature. The world seemed so much simpler then. We had the microscopes to find the problem-causing microbes, and the big guns—the antibiotics, the vaccines, the disinfectants—to kill the microbes or at least prevent them from causing disease. Smallpox had been defeated, and diseases such as polio and measles were lined up in the eradication queue. Other scourges such as leprosy and tuberculosis seemed to have just fled large parts of the world, leaving few explanations behind. The best bets for what got rid of them are better food, cleaner water, and good housing—nothing really spectacular, nothing to patent.

Globally, infectious diseases really did seem to have taken a holiday; most people are more likely to die from accidents, suicides, heart disease, or strokes than from infections. But the microbes are still there, as anybody not living in suburban enclaves in North America, Europe, and Australia could have told us. In a 1990 study of causes of death worldwide, heart disease and strokes were number one and number two, respectively, but right behind them were respiratory infections and diarrhea. The bugs are still out there.

In fact, the more scientists look, and the better the detection technology, the more microbes there seem to be. In the late seventeenth century, Anton Van Leeuwenhoek saw what he called "animalcules," tiny animals, through his microscopes. Now there are electron microscopes, which can take pictures not only of bacteria but also of viruses and even those impossible disease makers, the prions. Viruses are thin bits of DNA (deoxyribonucleic acid) or RNA (ribonucleic acid), covered with distinctive jackets of protein. They move long distances quickly. They are the ultimate cool, athletic anorexics. There are uncountable numbers of viruses jostling around. They get into a bloodstream through a nostril or a gut or by being mainstreamed through the good graces of a blood-feeding arthropod. Once inside, they take over the host cells and use the organism's machinery to reproduce themselves. Mostly, they shuffle and sneeze and poke their way around pretty quietly, bird to mosquito to bird to mosquito to mouse. Viruses are probably as old as the oldest ancestors of the animals they infect, so there has been a long time to co-evolve and learn how to be good neighbors. Usually no one gets hurt.

In the southern United States, west of the Mississippi, there is a virus called western equine encephalitis (WEE). The virus multiplies in the blood of a variety of birds and in certain mosquitoes (*Culex tarsalis*). The original homeland of the virus was in a community of marsh-dwelling mosquitoes and birds such as blackbirds and swallows. It lived there for a long time without causing any serious problems in the animals it infected. As people moved in and, through drainage, irrigation, and land cultivation, destroyed some of that habitat and modified what was left, the viruses and the birds adapted. The birds found new sources of food, such as grain in fields or in grain bins, and the viruses found new hosts with cells to hijack.

On the one hand, they needed some warm-blooded species with fast population turnover, so that there was always a fresh, non-immune crop to invade; house sparrows, which emigrated from Europe in the mid-nineteenth century, seem to fill that role in many areas. On the other hand, the viruses also needed mosquitoes willing to feed on both birds and mammals. With more than 150 species of mosquitoes in the United States (several thousand in the world), feeding at different times of day on a variety of species, everywhere from deep mine shafts to high mountains, the odds were pretty good that appropriate mosquito carriers could be found. The life cycle expanded so that WEE virus can now infect wild rodents, chickens, and pigs without, apparently, making them ill.

Not all animals have been so lucky. In the summer of 1930, about six thousand horses in the San Joaquin Valley, in California, came down with a mysterious brain disease. They became unco-ordinated, somnolent, and fatigued. Half of the horses died. The disease was WEE. From the 1930s to the 1970s, outbreaks and epidemics of WEE occurred in people and animals all through the western United States and north into Manitoba, Saskatchewan, and Alberta, in Canada; thousands of horses and hundreds of people got sick. Although birds and their attendant mosquitoes can maintain the virus in nature, mammals are apparently a so-called dead-end host: they can get the disease but usually don't get enough viruses in the blood to pass on.

From my memory of growing up in Winnipeg, Manitoba, hot, muggy weather, migratory birds, and great veils of mosquitoes drifting across the back lawn are staple features of the prairies. The question is not so much why the disease occurred, but why it didn't occur every year, and why it only attacked in some places and not others, when the birds and damned mosquitoes were everywhere. Could any of the outbreaks be predicted?

In the first instance, investigators used the fact that chickens get infected, and hence develop antibodies to WEE, without getting sick. For many years, putting cages of chickens outside in strategic locations and periodically collecting involuntary blood donations from them to look for antibodies provided an interesting way to anticipate a coming epidemic. Rainfall and temperature conditions could be used to project mosquito populations; as the number of mosquitoes, and, if the virus was present, the rate of infection in chickens, increased, the probability of a serious epidemic could also be anticipated. This kind of epidemic prediction required a fair amount of intensive monitoring and still left unanswered the big questions: where did the viruses come from before they got to the chickens, and could the disease be stopped or predicted earlier?

Did any of the patterns of this disease have to do with where the virus stayed in the winter? Where *did* it stay in the winter? When I was in veterinary college, our instructor, John Iverson, had us take Richardson's ground squirrels out of the walk-in cooler and watched them slowly wake up. Iverson, a scientist who could suddenly switch his costume and, it seemed, his personality, from a three-piece suit to a white laboratory coat to rugged field gear, had a theory that the virus overwintered in these abundant rodents. After all, they do harbor a whole lot of other microbes. In the spring, when the last dirty patches of snow disappeared and chunks of floating ice clogged up canals and creeks, mosquitoes came alive in puddles by the road and migrating birds arrived from the south, initiating a cycle of amplification. By the time lovers strolled bare-armed through the woods, leading their horses behind them, the mosquitoes were singing in the sweet prairie air, and the epidemics could start in earnest. Other scientists suggested that the virus overwintered in frogs or snakes or that it just lived through the winter in the gut of the hibernating mosquitoes (the way West Nile virus does).

At the time WEE was being investigated, researchers were asking the same questions about a similar, less common (a few cases a year in horses, at most) but more serious disease—eastern equine encephalitis (EEE). This one occurs sporadically from Louisiana north into Michigan, Ontario, Connecticut, and Quebec. It also appears to kill ring-necked pheasants and a few other birds as well as the occasional horse or person, but it is otherwise a little beast similar to the WEE virus.

One of the most plausible and intriguing theories is that these viruses don't overwinter in the north at all. Like many weary northerners, they spend the winter quietly reproducing in warm southern areas, along the Gulf Coast for WEE and Florida for EEE.

In the 1980s, two Canadian researchers, Robert Sellers and Abdel Marouf, published a series of papers in which they asked: between 1980 and 1983, did WEE-infected mosquitoes ride the wind currents up from the Gulf of Mexico into Manitoba, Minnesota, and North Dakota? They found that a northward movement of warm air, meeting a cold front with rain, could well have carried infected mosquitoes and then dropped them at various locales in stages as summer crept its way farther north. It is a difficult theory to prove absolutely, given that mosquitoes are hard to microchip and that unstable weather patterns, vaccination of horses, changing landscapes, and changing habits of people all contribute to transforming a probability into an event.

Still, I am reminded of the time I was working on developing an animal-disease-monitoring system in the Caribbean in the late 1980s. One of my colleagues called me into his office one day to show me a giant locust in a jar of alcohol on his desk. "It's an African locust," he said. "I picked it up on the beach, right here in Trinidad." He paused. "Thank God they don't have enough space to swarm here." One of the Trinidadian women laughed. "Typical," she said in her slow lilt. "The big males fly over and then just lie on the beach all day."

It occurred to me to wonder: if those big lugs can blow over from western Africa and flop down on the beach in Trinidad, how hard can it be for a mosquito infected with WEE to get from, say, Texas to Manitoba? This also occurred to me later, when West Nile virus exploded into North American consciousness. A lot of other individual events have to fall into a particular pattern for an epidemic like that of West Nile virus to occur, but with the ecological, climatic, and social world in constant, rapid flux, and nobody really paying very close attention, it was bound to happen sooner or later.

The long-term patterns of WEE, like those of so many other mosquito-borne viruses, are puzzling. Although St. Louis and eastern equine encephalitis both make their periodic, sporadic appearances, the once-feared widespread epidemics of western equine encephalitis have all but disappeared. The Centers for Disease Control and Prevention suggest that the intensity of the natural cycle for WEE increases every five to ten years, leading to a higher probability of epidemics, yet the last epidemic in horses or people was in 1987. But the lack of disease in horses shouldn't be a surprise.

We take care of our horses. There's money in doing so. Effective vaccines against equine encephalitis were developed quickly, advertised widely, and rapidly made available to veterinarians. There are no similar vaccines for people. Who would pay? Who bets on people running around a dirt track? Vaccines are good for the horses (and the vets and the people who make vaccines), but the antibodies produced by the vaccine often interfere with our ability to differentiate animals that got the real infection from those that were vaccinated. Furthermore, if horses are vaccinated, there is no use monitoring them for infection or disease, so where do researchers look to find out if the virus is still out there, looking for another opportunity? They can monitor the sentinel chickens and look for antibodies in them, and they can search for the virus in mosquitoes. But if there haven't been any cases of serious disease reported recently, there is less pressure on government agencies to maintain monitoring programs. Money gets directed to other priorities until the next outbreak occurs.

People tend to get sloppy about vaccination when the vaccine works and the disease disappears. It is a general problem of preventive health programs that if they are successful, nothing happens, so governments and individuals are always tempted to disinvest in the most successful of them. Why would a horse owner pay someone a lot of money to stick a needle into her horse if there's no disease around? In 1987, there was a northward wave of WEE from the Rio Grande; starting in April and continuing into June, the virus moved north through the Texas Panhandle, New Mexico, and Oklahoma; in July, it headed farther north across the Great Plains; by August, it was in North Dakota, Manitoba, and Minnesota. Thirty-seven people and 132 horses were reported sick. In the Imperial and Sacramento valleys of California, the sentinel chickens developed antibodies to the virus, demonstrating that it was in the wild mosquito and bird populations, but no horses or people got sick. The chickens are the scientific equivalent of omens, but what is the message? What should be done?

Some have suggested that not much WEE is seen anymore not just because people vaccinate their horses, but also because there have been aggressive programs for spraying against mosquitoes. Others have proposed that this disease, like many others, has succumbed to broader social changes. One study in California demonstrated that between 1945 and 1982, counties that had higher ownership of televisions and air conditioners were less likely to have cases of equine encephalitis than places where fewer people had these newfangled luxuries. Apparently folks are now inside at dusk, watching television sitcoms in air-conditioned comfort and arguing about what's for supper instead of playing ball with their kids at dusk or sitting on the porch reading a newspaper. Their horses, of course, are vaccinated. And nobody really cares about what's out there, cycling between birds and mosquitoes. But with increased air conditioning and more television sets comes increased energy use, which translates into longer-term climate change. I doubt that those birds, their viruses, and mosquitoes are done with us yet.

(7)

WEST NILE VIRUS

AND THE ST. LOUIS BLUES

WE HAD beer and chips at Jinja, where the Nile River flows out of Lake Victoria. We read the broken, rust-colored plaque there, amid the greenery near the steady flow of water where Rippon Falls used to be, before the Owen Falls Dam was built just downstream. The plaque proclaimed John Hanning Speke the discoverer of that most elusive and mysterious prize, the origin of the Nile. Still, I felt more pleasant tropical turpitude than historical grandeur. It was late May 2000. The place was quiet, just a few of the once-numerous Indian-Ugandan merchants and Western tourists starting to come back after the brutal ethnic cleansing of the Amin years.

A breeze wafted over us from the lake as a gray-headed kingfisher, with brilliant reddish-orange beak and strong blue and black wing markings, dropped down toward the water.

It was a place steeped in lovely natural vistas and pompous European views. The Arabs, looking for gold, ivory, and slaves, had produced the so-called Al Adrisi map of "Lake Victoria" (which was called Ukerewe until renamed in 1858) in the 1160s and described the lake as the source of the Nile. Ptolemy, that brilliant Alexandrian scholar, had more vague suggestions of lake sources of the Nile almost a thousand years before that. In the history of Western civilization, however, the lake's true iden-tity and the name and the origin of the Nile could not really be known until a European had named them appropriately.

The lake was renamed after Queen Victoria, and the name stuck. Wealthy and inexperienced British explorer John Speke, who was on an expedition with the legendary Richard Burton, upstaged his companion (while Burton was recovering from ill-ness) and proclaimed Lake Victoria the source of the Nile in 1858. Burton later challenged Speke to a debate over the true origins of the Nile before the Royal Geographical Society. Speke died just before the event in a mysterious hunting accident. A German, Dr. Burkhart Waldecker, trumped both of them by declaring in 1937 (from a safe temporal distance, since Burton and Speke were both dead by then) that the real source was a bubbling moun-tain spring in Burundi, or perhaps the Mountains of the Moon in Rwanda, fed by melting snows. Starting as snowmelt and spring water, the streams and creeks gather into small rivers, which eventually join to become the Nile. As climate change "disappears" the snow at the headwaters, one wonders what will become of the Nile.

North from where we sat on that day in May, the Victoria Nile tumbles and flows through lakes Kyoga and Albert and north into the slow, shimmering spread of the marshy Sudd in southern Sudan. Eventually, sluggishly and now known as the White Nile, it heads to Khartoum, where it joins the Blue Nile and then con-tinues its northern progress through ancient kingdoms and into world history. Looking north and east, we were facing country-side ravaged by sleeping sickness and war; to the north and west lay an area that, in America at least, had become famous in 1999 as the origins of the West Nile virus.

The virus was first isolated in 1937 from a febrile adult woman in the West Nile district of Uganda; in the 1950s, Egyptian researchers found it in mosquitoes, birds, and people. In 1957, in Israel, it was recognized as a cause of severe human inflammation of the spinal cord and brain. Over the next few decades, cases in people and horses were recognized throughout the western Mediterranean, southern Russia, and eastern and southern Europe.

Like the geographically and emotionally complicated Nile River, which pre-dated its "discoverers" by tens of thousands of years, the virus and the infection pre-dated its discovery by hundreds of millions of years. Some have now suggested that Alexander the Great may have died of West Nile virus; Babylon, where he died, was thick with mosquitoes, and ravens fell from the sky on the day of his death. Others believe that he more likely died of typhoid fever, a supposition that doesn't explain the falling ravens and is somewhat less interesting.

As long as West Nile virus kept its range to a variety of bird species, traveling regularly between Africa, Asia, the Middle East, and Europe, or to occasional cases in marginalized Africans, researchers, at least in North America, didn't pay a lot of attention. To be fair, although there was evidence of the virus and some very closely related ones (such as Kunjin, which is found in Australia and some South Pacific islands) just about everywhere in the world, infection in either the birds or people didn't usually have serious consequences. But it is a sign of the general biological narrow-mindedness of many medical researchers that they didn't see the summer of 1999 coming.

In that hot, dry summer of 1999 in New York City, people (and a variety of birds at the zoo) were getting sick, and some were dying, from an unidentified neurological disease. At first, medical investigators called it St. Louis encephalitis virus. Actually, at first they didn't call it anything; the disease was hardly noticed at all. Who would notice a few people dying of strange diseases in New York City? When they did call it St. Louis encephalitis, it sort of made sense.

St. Louis encephalitis had periodically caused similar outbreaks in the southern United States and was, until West Nile
virus came along, the most common cause of viral encephalitis
in the U.S. In 1999, there were twenty reported cases of St. Louis
encephalitis in New Orleans. That was about a typical year. In
the mid-1970s, an epidemic afflicting about 2,500 people over
thirty-five states was deemed by authorities to be an aberration.
Another epidemic in Colorado in the mid-1980s infected over a
thousand people, although fewer than two dozen reported being
sick; one person died.

That pattern of sporadic outbreaks and silent infections, in
which many people do not actually report being sick, is fairly
typical for a lot of these viruses. Since the mid-1960s and until
West Nile virus hit, there had been close to five thousand cases
of St. Louis encephalitis in the U.S. Epidemiologists looking for
patterns say that St. Louis encephalitis virus causes epidemics every ten or eleven years in the United States, apparently in
inverse synchronicity with sunspot activity. I don't think anyone
was actively monitoring sunspots in 1999.

The 1999 suspect cases in New York were a bit out of the usual
southwestern range for St. Louis encephalitis, but then so are a lot
of species these days, including us, so this shouldn't be a surprise.

Mosquito-borne members of the extended family of the genus
Flavivirus, to which West Nile virus belongs, may often only
cause aches and pains, but they can, and do, lead to all kinds of
neurological havoc in a small percentage of those who get sick.
Kunjin virus in Australia is usually associated with a mild disease in people, but Murray Valley encephalitis, which cycles naturally between birds (herons and pelicans) and mosquitoes, is
more often a life-threatening disease in people.

Japanese encephalitis, carried in pigs and wild birds in many
parts of Asia, is spread to people through mosquitoes. Mostly this
virus quietly cycles between pigs, birds, frogs, and mosquitoes,

but in pigs it can cause abortion and piglet death. The type of mosquito that transmits the virus seems to reproduce especially well in fertilized rice paddies. In people, the virus may cause anything from a few aches and pains and fever to bleeding from the gums and nose to full-blown seizures and death. Tens of thousands of people get sick from it in eastern Asia every year. One in five of these die. There is a vaccine, which works pretty well.

Among all this family of diseases, the one most vigorously and seriously investigated has been yellow fever, probably because it was of interest to the U.S. military. In its home in tropical Africa, yellow fever cycles naturally between mosquitoes that breed in holes in trees and tropical forest primates. The disease itself can be quite awful. With its bleeding from various orifices, bloody vomit, and yellowing of the skin from liver damage, we might understand why port cities in the eighteenth and nineteenth centuries did not welcome ships attempting to enter port carrying sailors afflicted with what they called yellow jack.

Through our incorrigible meddling and bad luck, we not only managed to bring the virus to the Western Hemisphere but also managed to select for a species of the carrier mosquito, *Aedes aegypti*, that bred in holes in "horizontal trees," that is, in water tanks on slave ships. In tropical America, the disease caused considerable devastation for a couple of hundred years and settled into new niches, both urban and sylvatic. It killed 27,000 of Napoleon's best troops in the Caribbean and opened the door for Haitian independence. A Cuban physician, Carlos Finlay, carefully hypothesized that the disease was transmitted by mosquitoes, a finding that was confirmed by the U.S. army surgeon Walter Reed in 1901. The discovery of what spread the disease (mosquitoes) and how to control it (mosquito netting on beds, cleaning up standing water) gave the American troops an edge in their conquest of tropical America, including the ability to build the Panama Canal. Today the disease occurs as a human-mosquito-human disease in poor urban tropical areas, and as a zoonosis for those who have unprotected intercourse with certain tropical rain forests.

The World Health Organization suggests that 200,000 people get yellow fever annually, and 30,000 of them die. Again, there's a good vaccine, and the fact that people are still getting sick and dying has more to do with social and economic justice than with a paucity of science. Only a few people, like myself, can't take the vaccine because they are allergic to eggs; the vaccine (like that for influenza) is based on growing the virus in eggs.

Okay, so the deaths in New York were not yellow fever or Japanese encephalitis. Even the West Nile thing seemed a bit of a zebra. But what if the hoofbeats you hear in New York City *are*, against considerable odds, those of a zebra? What if it is a virus from Africa and the Middle East? What if we live in the twenty-first century, when we are juggling and shipping and smuggling microbes around the world in agricultural produce and exotic pets and traveling relatives just about as fast as we can? Then you might be caught with your intellectual pants down.

After the genetic and antigenic mapping of viruses from a dead flamingo, a couple of people, and some mosquitoes, using envelope-glycoprotein-specific monoclonal antibodies (meaning they tested specifically for the proteins on the outside of the virus), the disease was confirmed to indeed be due to infection with West Nile virus. Not only that, but investigators could say with some certainty that it was related to one isolated from a dead goose in Israel in 1998 (ah, that I were so sure of my own relatives). By the end of that summer of 1999, more than sixty people were reported sick, and seven died, from the disease. A later investigation suggested that the number of people infected might have been over eight thousand. As is usual when we first stumble across a new disease (or it stumbles across us), we only noticed the most serious cases.

That initial outbreak of what has turned into a continent-wide epidemic has spawned more versions and stories than actual cases of disease, which should tell us something about scientists, how science is really done, and how we might learn our way through the complex challenges of life in the twenty-first century. But I will come back to that at the end of the book. For West Nile virus in North America, there were the usual stories of the medico-political soap opera variety, as well as ecological morality tales, whispers of plots and Jewish travelers, and great public health and biotechnological successes.

Some wondered what would have happened if arrogant health officials at the Centers for Disease Control and Prevention hadn't discounted the information from a (female) veterinarian that birds (Crows! Who cares?) were dying in New York City. By most accounts, Tracey McNamara, the veterinarian at the Bronx Zoo who was studying a substantial die-off of birds in the area, was apparently sidelined, ignored, and shabbily treated by the single-species-trained medical investigators even as she gathered the evidence needed to unravel the nature of the mystery agent. The number of cowboy egos riding around at the Centers for Disease Control and Prevention amazed some outsiders, but probably not those who are used to the Byzantine world of competitive science, inside and outside academia. In much of Canada, collegiality and teamwork tends to prevail over cutthroat competition, but, not to be too smug, much good scientific work in Canada has also been stifled by kow-towing to corporate or other ideologies and an intransigent refusal by many government departments to share information. Whether any of these shenanigans made any difference in the outcome is hard to say, since by the time the spraying for mosquitoes started, the epidemic was mostly over.

Some suggested that the West Nile virus outbreak was a bioterrorist attack by a shadowy group of freedom fighters trying to bring down the Empire. Hadn't the most recently reported outbreak, killing about fifty of five hundred people affected, been in Romania? Wasn't there also an outbreak in southern Russia, before the crows started dying in New York? There was. As the political activist Abbie Hoffman once said, "Just because you're paranoid doesn't mean they are not out to get you." Or maybe the outbreak was just a message from our old friends the migrating birds, who return each year to remind us that we are part of a global ecosystem (which we, as often as not, then quickly forget). Certainly, the New York outbreak was in an area near wetlands frequented by migrating birds, mosquitoes, and people.

But once the virus was here, it was here. After that first summer, it seemed to lie low, getting a foothold: the right mosquitoes, the right birds, the right neighborhoods. Climate change had no doubt made North America more hospitable to a virus that must surely have visited our shores before: warmer winters allowing better mosquito survival, drought and heat bringing birds and mosquitoes closer together at pools of water (where they build up high levels of virus), followed by heavy rains that cause them to fan out over wide geographic areas. Whatever the reasons, the virus found a home, settled in for a year or so, and then, in good biblical fashion, multiplied and spread. In 2000, there were 29 human cases in the U.S.; in 2001, 666; in 2002, over 4,000; and the following year, almost 10,000. The numbers reflected a great wave moving across the continental United States and Canada. Interestingly, behind the wave, the numbers settled. In the U.S., there were 2,500 cases in 2004, and just under 3,000 in 2005.

In Canada, sick birds first showed up in 2001, and human cases started appearing in 2002, at which time Ontario's medical officer of health publicly dismissed West Nile as being trivial compared with the annual influenza epidemic that swept across North America. This statement did not endear him to the worried public but raised some interesting questions. Should the importance of diseases be judged by the number of cases? Number of deaths? Disability-adjusted life years? The population affected? *E. coli* 0157:H7 had affected many thousands of people with minimal social impact before it hit a few middle-class children, at which time it transformed the entire American meat inspection system. Are diseases that surprise us more important than diseases we have come to take for granted? Surprise, after all, indicates that either scientists are in the dark or they haven't been watching carefully enough in the right places. Surprise (more cases than "expected") is one of the key elements in an epidemic.

The first year, diagnoses were made slowly in Ontario because no one seemed prepared, although, based on tracking of possible paths the epidemic would take, investigators had a couple of years' notice. But the tracking came from those animal-disease people, and what do they know? This wasn't the flu, after all. Early reports suggested there were fewer than a hundred human cases that first year; later reports suggested closer to four hundred. In 2003, West Nile virus took flight westward across the country—or, more probably, having flown south from the eastern seaboard, the virus moved north on a new flight path. More than a thousand cases occurred in the Prairie provinces, and the disease spilled over the mountains to the West Coast. Birds, after all, fly, and many of the infected birds were returning from the southern United States, where the disease was already quite nicely settling into its New World habitat.

And everywhere, crows, ravens, magpies, and jays were dropping dead. Most of the dead birds were corvids, but not all of them. In Ontario, an outbreak in an owl rehabilitation center killed off most of the larger, northern-breeding owls but left many of the smaller, southern-breeding owls alone. In that colony, which was designed to rehabilitate injured birds and release them to the wild, the virus appeared to be transmitted by the biting louse fly. It is doubtful that the virus was transmitted to animals or people outside the colony. Most people tend not to get close to owls, but veterinary students can get weird that way.

When I was in veterinary college, I spent part of a summer helping to retrain injured and repaired owls before they were returned to the wild. As part of the retraining, they would sit on my arm and then chase dead mice that someone threw. Partway through the summer, I started getting severe headaches, and my memory was affected. One day my sister-in-law telephoned, and, after a cheery but apparently strange conversation with her, I hung up and promptly forgot that she had called. When my wife figured out that something was wrong, she drove me to the hospital; I then spent many weeks in bed getting delirious, hallucinating, and suffering splitting headaches from what was diagnosed as viral meningitis. We suspected the owls, but it could have been a dozen other exposures.

Owls can carry *Chlamydophila psittaci*, the microbe that causes parrot fever. The organism used to be called *Chlamydia psittaci*, but the name was changed, in part to reflect new genetic information; the change also serves to clear up the confusion between this zoonotic chlamydial infection and the chlamydia that cause vaginal infections in people. Psittacosis in people can range from a mild respiratory infection to fever, chills, and serious pneumonia, but people more often pick that up from breathing aerosolized feces of pet birds. In the United States in 2005, there was an outbreak of salmonellosis among elementary school children who had dissected owls' fecal pellets. Despite these few possibilities, the cases of actual transmission are really few. During the peaks of the West Nile virus epidemic, dying or dead hawks, pheasants, and other birds that were suffering from the disease were also being taken in to wildlife disease investigation centers around North America.

Crows and ravens have historically been birds with messages, often dark ones. In this case, some people thought that the messenger might be the message, that crows were carrying the virus that was going to kill us all. A virus that kills so many of its reservoir host, however, wouldn't last long; this is Darwinian selection at its simplest. One continuing question in West Nile virus investigations is where the virus has been making its home when it wasn't out on killing sprees or instilling fear into suburbanites. Who *wasn't* it killing?

In 2004, Sharon Calvin, a veterinarian doing graduate studies under my supervision, decided to investigate a possible candidate for harboring West Nile virus: gulls. The Leslie Street Spit is the eastern headland of a three-mile-long peninsula extending from the Toronto shoreline into Lake Ontario. Now a home to a park and wildlife refuge, the peninsula has been built up from harbor dredge and industrial waste over fifty years. In early summer, as one stands at the edge of the spit before a heaving sea of squawking and yelling and crying birds amid flying feathers, with feces and urine spraying across the heat-edged sky, it is difficult to imagine a time that gulls were ever endangered.

As with so many other species, humans destroyed gulls' early abundance through destruction of habitat and use of feathers for hats and eggs for food. From huge numbers in the early 1800s, ring-billed gulls all but disappeared from the Great Lakes Basin by the beginning of the next century. Then, in 1917, Canada, the United States, Mexico, and Russia signed the Migratory Birds Convention Act. Those who doubt the effectiveness of such governmental agreements need only visit the Toronto waterfront. The agreement was aided by the provision of an abundant food supply for these garbage-eating omnivores and the creation of new nesting sites made of concrete, slag, mud, and other so-called wastes left in the wake of city building. Gulls, at least, benefited from this protection; there are now probably three-quarters of a million nests in the Great Lakes Basin and upper St. Lawrence River.

So, in 2004, there they were, multiplying as fast as we could feed them and provide habitat. And not dying from West Nile virus. We already knew that gulls, like Canada geese, another species to benefit from waterfowl protection, can pick up all kinds of gut-wrenching human pathogens from garbage dumps and farm manure (*Salmonella* and *Campylobacter,* for instance) and then spread them around to new places. We knew that bird (and bat) guano is an excellent medium for *Histoplasma capsulatum,* a fungus that, once inhaled, turns into a yeast and causes pneumonia in people, but that is a risk for people cleaning up old buildings, not for the general public. We knew that gulls can carry some strains of Newcastle disease virus, first discovered in Indonesia and England in the 1920s and now known to be a worldwide killer of domestic chickens. The virus is a member of the family *Paramyxoviridae,* which includes the viruses that cause measles and mumps, as well as the zoonotic Hendra and Nipah viruses (see chapter 9); in its most pathogenic form, Newcastle disease has devastated poultry farms around the world. More recently, another strain has killed cormorants and pelicans in North America. In people (mostly veterinarians and poultry farmers), Newcastle disease causes conjunctivitis and headaches.

Being waterbirds, gulls also carry a variety of avian influenza viruses. An outbreak of avian influenza had killed a few hundred gulls living like vagabonds on a rooftop in my hometown, Kitchener-Waterloo, Ontario, and an earlier study had found evidence of avian influenza virus (H13N6, if you want the numbers) in almost all the 360 gulls tested from colonies on Lake Ontario. Well, waterbirds are the natural home of influenza viruses, so this should not have been a big surprise. Why not West Nile virus?

In the summer of 2004, residents of Toronto and Hamilton could see small teams of people in white space suits and hard hats (to protect them against dive-bombing, shit-spraying birds) chasing gulls with nets in the wild reaches of the Leslie

Street Spit and the shores of Hamilton Harbour. Throughout the summer, Sharon worked with our team at the University of Guelph and the Public Health Agency of Canada, bleeding and swabbing mothers and chicks and trapping mosquitoes.

It turned out to be a great year for the public and a bad year to look for West Nile virus. We found evidence of the other two viruses Sharon was looking for, but neither the mosquitoes nor the birds came up positive for West Nile virus. It could have been the cooler summer, the government mosquito-control programs, the design of the study, or the tests we used, or it could be that gulls are not a big part of the West Nile virus story. That's science.

Many researchers now think that songbirds such as American robins carry the virus without getting sick, perhaps because they are more likely to hang around in mosquito-ey neighborhoods. There has also been a suggestion that alligators could be important amplifiers of the disease, although that would have been unlikely in New York and very unlikely in southern Ontario.

Besides birds, the virus needs mosquitoes to get around. As with WEE and other mosquito-borne diseases, a variety of mosquito populations are involved in maintaining and spreading West Nile. Some mosquitoes keep it going among birds, and others spread it from birds to people. From the human point of view, mosquitoes sometimes seem indiscriminate in their thirst for blood. In fact, not all mosquitoes are out to get us; most mosquitoes (all the males) are nectar feeders. There is even one species, the toxorhynchites, sometimes called mosquito hawks, whose larvae feed on the larvae of other mosquitoes.

AFTER A GREAT wave of money, panic, and scientific work, interest in West Nile virus subsided. The virus is here, quietly circulating in its newfound home, periodically making people and animals sick. Except for those unfortunate few who suffered the neurological form of the disease—and for those people, it is and will always be a tragedy—life has continued. If, in West Nile virus, nature was reminding us of our mortality, of our kinship with bacteria, viruses, birds, and mosquitoes, and of the integral part of tragedy in the human condition, then we have brushed that reminder aside. But nature will not so easily be dismissed. In 2006, even as West Nile virus was dropping off the public radar screen, North Americans discovered a new bird-related disease about which to panic and which is the subject of the next chapter: avian influenza.

(8)

THE CHICKENS FIGHT BACK

*T*HE BRIGHT, fierce, piercing cry startled me from sleep. Groggily, bathed in sweat, I pushed away my Dutch wife—that long, cylindrical pillow so beloved in all traditional Javanese hotels. In one stumbling motion, I swung out of bed, pulled my sarong around my waist, ran to the door, and stuck my head outside into the misty tropical air. Several yards away, on a low branch, perched the regal father of all chickens. His wattles were full, fleshy, and pink. Like the robes of some strutting bird-king, his cape flowed down from his crown, over his back, in brilliant bronze, rust, and gold, ending in a ruff of white. His lower chest and fountaining tail feathers shimmered in the early morning sunlight from deep black to blue to green. His sharp black eye caught mine and held it. This was not a bird to quietly back down from a challenge.

The red jungle fowl, and its gray and green siblings, was first domesticated in South and eastern Asia—India, Myanmar, Thailand, Laos, Vietnam, China, Malaysia, Java—many thousands of years ago. These birds were originally bred for cockfighting. From India, the birds explored westward into Persia, carrying with them their wild spirit, and, one assumes, the populations of viruses and bacteria living in their intestines. There is no evidence that they were considered a low-fat, low-cost, low-carb food or a public health threat.

The Zoroastrians praised cocks for driving out the devils of night and guarding the household. From Persia, the birds invaded both northern Africa and Europe. Although the "rosy-fingered Dawn" Homer described in *The Odyssey* was not accompanied by cockcrows, Aeschylus (late in the fifth century BC) has Athena (in the play *The Eumenides*) warning the Greeks that civil war is like cockfighting, an image (fierce, small-brained, beautiful birds passionately slashing each other to death) that some of us would extend to war in general, although cockfighting itself has perhaps more to recommend it.

The Romans used live chickens for augurs; if the birds eagerly ate food thrown to them, things would go well. If not, this was a poor omen. As might be expected, the chickens were kept underfed until omen-reading time came around. During a 249 BC battle against the Carthaginians at Drepana, in what is now western Sicily, the Roman consul P. Claudius Pulcher threw the sacred chickens overboard when they refused to eat, saying, "If they will not eat, let them drink." Later the same day, the Carthaginians sank 93 of the consul's 123 ships. The consul was promptly recalled and forced to pay a large fine. One could draw a lesson from this event, but it would be premature for me to pronounce omens so early in this story.

Later on that 1986 morning in Java, sipping my jasmine tea and nibbling on sweet buns, I watched a scattering of various-sized *kampung* ("village") chickens scratching through the dirt between the buildings, under the banana, mango, and jackfruit trees, skittering out from under the wheels of predatory buses and trucks roaring by in clouds of dirty diesel on the nearby asphalt highway. A woman leaning forward on her motorcycle, a feathery bustle of chickens hung by their claws and flouncing out behind her, snarled past, heading to market. The rust and black feathers of the *kampung* birds, although thin and shabby by comparison with those of their wild cousins, still showed traces of royal blood.

In the late 1980s, in the local markets of Java, *kampung* chicken brought a premium price compared with the amount paid for their fast-growing, placid urban cousins. So precious were they that nothing was wasted. Our family dined at Nyonya Suharti's, Java's answer to KFC, in Yogyakarta, in the province of Central Java. The pieces were tasty, very tender, and finger-licking greasy.

"You know," our nine-year-old son said, "in this country, some people eat the chicken heads and everything."

I already knew about, and had tried, the curried soup made with chicken intestines. I looked at the batter-smothered piece of bird I had just set down and recognized a beak, a comb, and an eye. The brain was already eaten away—by me. Everyone at the table laughed uproariously at my lack of attention to what I had been eating.

"That's something to write home about," laughed my wife, Kathy.

"The brain tasted like liver," I said.

Kathy looked down at her plate, at the piece she had just finished: a beak, a comb, an eye, the brain eaten away.

"I wondered what that was," she said.

Eating the brains of chickens does not have the same moral or infectious-disease baggage that eating monkey brains does (see chapter 10). Still, even for someone who was, when faced with some straggling bits of dinner left on the plate, reminded about the starving children of India, the idea that some cultures really do take to heart the adage "Waste not, want not" can be disconcerting. And if there was no waste at the dinner end, neither was there waste at the farm end. Unlike their urban cousins, the village birds were fed nothing except scraps, required no extra building investments, and provided for their human neighbors' food, entertainment, and a sense of wonder at the beauty and cleverness of these silly birds.

Sometimes, as I drove through the country for my veterinary epidemiological work, I would pull over beside the narrow asphalt road to watch a line of ducks following a thin man, who carried a white flag flapping atop a bamboo staff. The man would have started from East Java, so I was told, with tiny ducklings. They would be imprinted on the white flag, following it like the dutiful, small-brained beauties that they are. The duck herder would stop at the watery muck of a recently harvested rice field, where the ducks would forage all day. At night, they would gather in a close flock around the white flag, for sleep and protection. The next day, they would walk on to another field, farther west.

Walking or swimming in roadside ditches, foraging in recently harvested rice fields, they would make their way to Jakarta, far to the west, where the ducks would be sold. The herder would take his money, ride the train back to his home in the east, and start over. Not a bad life, I thought, for the ducks and the herder. Good ecologically, good economically. And good, it turns out, for at least some of the viruses and bacteria that make their homes in bird poop.

A few years later, I stood in a broiler barn, that is, a barn where chickens are grown for meat, in southern Ontario. In my plastic boots and white throwaway safety suit (to protect the birds, not me) and a face mask (to keep the fine particles of litter-dust out of my lungs), I gazed out over ten thousand identical birds. The room was spacious and the litter was clean. Delivery of food, water, and air was computer controlled. The birds were white-feathered, plump, and only mildly curious about life. These were urban, office-dwelling birds. In five weeks, they could grow—uniformly, all of them—to the exact size required by KFC.

By the wonders of genetics and intensive breeding for specific traits, the fiercely wild stock of the jungle fowl had been transformed into something that could grow faster, more uniformly, and, by some standards, more efficiently. There was a chicken of identical size in every KFC pot. And if the genetic stock, the feed, and sometimes even the buildings were imported, and underpaid local labor used in place of underpriced fossil fuel, this feat could be accomplished just about anywhere in the world. This, too, is something amazing.

By 2006, the world was producing more than 88 million tons of chicken every year. The fastest growth in commercial poultry production was in the developing world. By the late 1990s, countries such as Indonesia and Brazil were increasing their commercial production by about 10 percent a year. China, already one of the world's biggest producers, was increasing at about 4 percent annually in the 1990s. Chickens were being grown, trucked, shipped, and fried as fast as the technology allowed. Who would have thought that so many people on this planet could be fed with such apparent ease? Who would have thought that this feat would also create the perfect conditions for barn-sized outbreaks—thousands of uniformly susceptible animals gathered under one roof—and then fit so neatly into a globally integrated system that created perfect conditions for a pandemic? Who would have thought human beings were so clever, and so naive?

But in ecology—which is to say, in a world where everything is, sooner or later, connected to everything else—there are costs, and trade-offs. By the end of the twentieth century, epidemiologists who specialize in food-borne diseases were already well aware that a pandemic of salmonellosis, a disease with both immediate effects on the gastrointestinal system and long-term effects on arthritis and cardiovascular disease, was one of the hidden costs of mass producing chicken (see my book *Food, Sex and Salmonella* for more on that).

This pandemic could have been taken as a warning, an omen from the chickens of the world, a shot across the bow, as it were. The omen was not cryptic. It might have been something like: the economies of scale for chicken production are the same as the economies of scale for disease; small farms have outbreaks; big farms breed epidemics; globalization of big farms creates pandemics. But, like Pulcher 2,200 years previously, humanity ignored the omen, threw the birds overboard, and put its faith in advances in food safety technology.

The omen having been ignored, few researchers in the late twentieth century would have stood in a chicken broiler barn and made the mental connections to ducks flying overhead, or to the populations of viruses and bacteria and parasites to whom the ducks are a quiet, comfortable vehicle for long-distance air travel. A few North American veterinarians, on thinking about ducks, might worry about them carrying the Newcastle disease virus that affects poultry, or the schistosome parasite that causes swimmers' itch or duck itch in people. These schistosomes normally cycle from waterfowl through open water to snails and back out through open water to birds or muskrats. Unlike their cousins *Schistosoma japonicum* in Southeast Asia, which can cause serious harm, these parasites don't actually like people. Their dives into human skin cause an allergic reaction and are kamikaze nosedives into itchy oblivion. But I digress.

That same week, after visiting the broiler barn, I stood outside in crisp fall sunshine next to the riffling waters of a beautiful Ontario marsh with a group of veterinary students learning about ecosystem health. In the crook of my arm, nestled on her back, was a wild mallard duck. I was swabbing her cloaca, the common passage where urine and feces come out. We were checking her for influenza virus, as part of a mock influenza outbreak.

Influenza viruses are simple, tiny things: eight segments of ribonucleic acid, or RNA, packed into a string or sphere about

80 to 100 nanometers in diameter (think billionths of meters; a hair shaft is about 100,000 nanometers, a bacterium about 1,000). Being small, they can get away with stuff bigger things cannot. They can reproduce without being alive, for instance; to reproduce, they commandeer the machinery of a living cell. Once inside, they are sloppily promiscuous, sharing bits and pieces, it seems, with whoever happens to be around. These viruses, classified as types A, B, and C, circulate in people, pigs, horses, birds, mink, and marine mammals. Type A is further subdivided into HA (hemagglutinin, of which there are at least sixteen types) and NA (neuraminidase) antigens (projections that stick out of the lipid envelope surrounding the RNA; there are about nine types of these).

As with personality types in people, type A is the most worrisome to health workers. The many different combinations of the virus genes vary almost infinitely in their ability to cause disease, which depends not just on the virus itself but on the genetic, health, and nutritional status, and on the organizational structure, of the populations into which they are introduced. The combination that was creating the greatest anxiety around the world in 2006 was H5N1 (hemagglutinin type 5, neuramidase type 1); although it is not easily transmitted, when it does transmit to other birds, to cats, to people, and to a variety of other species, it is unusually lethal. Influenza viruses are not supposed to behave this badly.

Waterbirds such as geese and ducks were domesticated even before jungle fowl, probably in the "cradle of civilization," the Middle East. Their intestines are the natural home for all sixteen known subtypes of influenza A viruses. You can test waterfowl of all sorts—ducks, geese, gulls—just about anywhere in the world and find some variations of them. Sharon Calvin found evidence of influenza infection in 80 percent of gulls in Toronto and Hamilton; many of the ducks we swabbed at that marsh as part of the mock influenza pandemic also harbored influenza viruses. It would have been surprising not to find them. For the most part, these influenza viruses in waterbirds are evolutionarily adapted and don't cause any disease problems in their natural hosts. However, when waterfowl are mixed with chickens and pigs and people in close quarters—as my ecologically friendly farmer friends were doing in Southeast Asia—novel opportunities for the viruses are created, they become genetically more unstable, and evolution is accelerated.

In 1996, a precursor of the H5N1 virus killed some geese in southern China. No one paid much attention. Then the virus picked up some gene fragments from quail and ducks, spread to the poultry markets in Hong Kong, and made the leap to humans; it killed six of eighteen people who were infected. Mass killing of all the domestic poultry in Hong Kong temporarily stopped the problem, but the virus continued to infect ducks and geese and to happily, sloppily evolve. In late 2002, a new variation of the virus killed off most of the waterfowl in Hong Kong nature parks. In the next few years, the new, more lethal variant spread through Vietnam, Thailand, Indonesia, Cambodia, Laos, China, Malaysia—the whole regional market. Not only was it making birds sick and killing them, but it was also infecting cats and ferrets and, finally, people.

When I lived in Indonesia in the 1980s, farming appeared to be an agro-ecologist's dream—lots of diversity, recycling of resources, low energy inputs. Influenza was a disease of people that periodically emerged from the creative microbial populations of southern China and wafted around the world, killing (mostly) older, already-debilitated people but generally leaving both non-human animals and the fit of our own species unscathed. Biodiversity in agriculture was seen as a solution, not a problem. So what happened?

Most commentators on the current global spread of influenza refer to the global pandemic of 1918, but the stories go back much farther than that. Hippocrates recorded an epidemic in 412 BC, and the name "influenza" itself comes from fifteenth-century Italy, referring to unexpected epidemics believed to be under the influence (influenza) of the stars. Not surprisingly, given the origins of chickens themselves, the first epidemic for which there is reasonably good information appears to have originated in Asia, before spreading to Africa and Europe. So ducks and chickens have been hanging around each other for a long time, and some kinds of influenza viruses have caused problems for as long as we can, collectively, remember. We learned to adjust; we monitored where the viruses came from (mostly southern China) and created vaccines. For most of the last century, these practices have kept matters more or less under control.

In May and June of 2005, one of the new variants of H5N1 killed more than five thousand wild bar-headed geese, gulls, and ducks in Qinghai Lake, China. Before they died, the affected birds had trouble standing and developed neurological problems (flopping around). Many researchers were worried that migratory birds would carry the virus down flyways into India. It looks as if they may have indeed carried the virus to Europe and Africa, but the evidence will always be ambiguous, and the world trade in poultry, both official and unofficial, remains an alternative explanation for how the disease has spread. To transport the virus, the wild birds have to be alive; if it is killing them, they stay where they are. If they survive, it could be because they have developed immunity or because the virus has evolved into something less pathogenic. In August 2006, the same virus turned up in cats in northern Iraq; so, however it was being transported and however dangerous it might be, it was certainly off to see the world.

Migratory birds carry all kinds of influenza viruses around the world, but the strains they carry usually don't kill them. If they are dying, it is likely because they are picking up new strains, which have evolved in domestically farmed populations. Another likely means of dissemination for the viruses we fear most is through the trucking of domestic and exotic birds around various continents—in other words, by people.

Some methods of spread are very culture-specific. In Thailand, fighting cocks are highly valued, reminding us of the origins of these birds as fighters. At matches, those betting money may go around and blow into the beaks of the contenders to check for lung capacity. Owners may suck mucus out through the beak between rounds. Traveling from match to match around the countryside, combined with this intimate contact, makes the fighting circuit a prime means of spreading the disease.

In October 2004, a Thai man flew into the Brussels airport from Bangkok with two crested hawk-eagles (*Spizaetus nipalensis*) in his hand luggage. He told customs officers they were for a friend. The birds, wrapped in cloth, stuffed into wicker tubes, and kept in the bag with the zipper left partly open for air, seemed healthy. They were "humanely sacrificed" (a very appropriate use of the term, since they gave their lives for the perceived greater good), and scientists looked for Newcastle disease and avian influenza. They found not only influenza but also the H5N1 strain that everyone feared. This kind of illegal trade is a huge business and a marvelous opportunity for all kinds of bacteria and viruses to find new homes in new lands.

Millions of tons of biological material—human food, animal feeds, meat-and-bone meal (MBM, which is basically animal offal reinvented as fertilizer for flowers in Indonesia, supplements for cats in America, and a variety of other essentials of modern life)—circle the globe annually. Economically, this circulation is described as free trade. Scientifically, it is simply carrying various types of living and non-living things from their ecological homes, where they usually cause few problems, to new areas, where they are very likely to cause a lot of problems. MBM was a major vehicle for transmitting bovine spongiform encephalopathy (BSE, or mad cow disease) within and between countries. One might be curious to know whether those who carefully crafted the documents of the World Trade Organization considered this possibility. One might wonder how many of them had some rudimentary knowledge of biology or even knew where food came from.

The farmers of Southeast Asia didn't scale up their production and increase the volume and speed of their trade in poultry products just "because"; they were responding to market demands for low-cost animal food. They are making a living by providing the protein and other nutrients that are necessary to sustain urban life; those farmers are, in a real sense, an essential part of the urban ecosystem. Without rapid economic growth and urbanization, avian influenza would likely remain a minor problem.

According to the United Nations, one in three people lived in a city in 1960. By the end of the twentieth century, almost half of all people did; by 2030, more than 60 percent of the population is expected to live in cities. Many of these megacities are in the developing world, especially in South and eastern Asia. These urban people want to eat, and they want protein. Chicken, ducks, geese, and pigs, all grown on an industrial model, will do just fine. Brazil, the United States, China, and the European Union are the world's biggest poultry producers. China leads the world in ducks and geese. Not surprisingly, other countries in the region—Thailand in particular—wanted to take advantage of these expanding urban markets and jumped into the hot economic fray. In places such as Thailand and Indonesia, increased production has sometimes been achieved by taking the kinds of laid-back, no-input chicken rearing I saw in the 1980s and scaling it up. If some chickens and ducks, mixed with rice paddies and fish ponds, are good, why aren't more better? Also not surprisingly, the current epidemic of avian influenza started in south China and has spread outward from there.

Still, the temptation to blame the wild birds, and not our own hubris, is strong.

When H5N1 appeared in Russia, rumors circulated that hunters were offering to shoot ducks to prevent the spread of the disease. Westerners laughed at this primitive response.

In October 2005, when cases of H5N1 influenza started appearing in Europe, British hunters stood at the ready, assured that shooting ducks was no mere macho hobby but an act of national public health importance, a serious form of scientific surveillance.

That same month the president of the United States gave the only response he seemed capable of imagining, saying he would rally the armed forces to fight the dreaded bird flu.

My friends who study wildlife suspect that the wild birds are picking it up from the domestic birds.

People who study viruses have pointed out that the H5 type of influenza virus found in China and a highly pathogenic H5N1 isolated from poultry in Scotland in 1959 share a common ancestor. Because influenza viruses are constantly drifting (small changes) and shifting (large, abrupt changes), the currently circulating strains are different from those first isolated. However, it would be disingenuous to suggest that intensification and global genetic "homogenization" of poultry production have not been driving forces in a variety of epidemics, including this one.

Some pontificators have suggested that farmers in South and eastern Asia should raise chickens the way we do in North America and Europe—inside tightly controlled buildings. These people have never lived in poor countries in the humid tropics, nor do they understand the systemic ramifications of creating a few large farms where once there were many small ones. If they want biosecurity such as we have in Europe and North America, the tropical farmers will need to close off the barns. But in the tropics, without air conditioning, the birds will start to die within minutes. With what power source would they air-condition? And what would happen to all those poor farmers in the countryside who depend on small flocks of poultry for food and to pay their school and medical bills? In the 1970s and 1980s, when we marveled at the man with the white flag and his ducks, the village chickens, and the wonder of the wild jungle fowl, were we off base? I think not. We've learned some things since then, and one of them, surely, must have something to do with the amazing complexity of the world we live in.

In 2005, the Millennium Ecosystem Assessment, an unprecedented global scientific effort to assess the world's ecosystems, demonstrated all the services that intact ecosystems provide for us—air, water, food, meaningful work—and just how vulnerable we all now are, with water and soils and forests and oceans at or near tipping points. No, if we want to find a solution to the influenza problem, more of the same won't cut it. Even if we kill all the sick chickens and put the rest into air-conditioned hotels, there will still be ducks flying overhead or cats or ferrets slinking in and out of the shrubbery. Some of the largest outbreaks of avian influenza have been in some of the best-managed poultry operations in the world, in some of the wealthiest countries. The viruses, like all microbes, adapt quickly to new situations. Already in late 2006, a new variation of the H5N1 avian influenza virus had emerged in China, possibly in response to selection pressures from vaccines given to chickens.

People in cities need food, but they need to be educated about where food comes from and the real costs of producing, processing, and shipping it. The energy costs of commercial chicken production, for instance, cannot be simply reduced to intake over output and then compared to cows, as is sometimes done. In this context, chicken always appears more efficient than other animal meats. But how much energy is required for the buildings and machinery, for growing special feeds, for getting the feed to the farm and the chickens to market? If the small farmers lose chickens as a source of livelihood, how will they pay for education and health care? All of these are real costs, which someone is paying.

Knowledge of the social and ecological dimensions of food should be part of every food consumer's education. An inability to prepare food and to talk intelligently about where that food comes from should be grounds for dismissal of politicians and corporate heads. And rather than circling the wagons in industrialized countries, we should see the threat of an avian influenza pandemic as our chance to work with farmers in poor southern countries to find complicated, low-energy ways of farming and to create a global animal-and-human health system accessible to everyone, everywhere. The ducks flying overhead are not a threat. They are a reminder.

One day, in 1986, I arrived at the veterinary college in Yogyakarta, Java, to find rows of very tall bamboo poles swaying in the slight breeze. At the top of each pole was a cage, and in each cage, a rooster. The proud birds were there to be judged on the quality of their calls; I do not know the criteria used by the judges, but standing there in the slight cool of a shady tropical morning, I could understand, like the Zoroastrians, how the calls of those jungle fowl might drive away the devils of darkness.

And Things That Go Bump in the Night

DISEASES PEOPLE GET

from ANIMALS, INVOLVING BATS

and RATS *but* NOT INSECTS

(9)

OUT OF NOWHERE:

NIPAH VIRUS AND SEVERE ACUTE

RESPIRATORY SYNDROME

NIPAH

In the first week of October 1994, I received an electronic message from ProMED, a fledgling international electronic bulletin board on emerging infectious diseases. Field workers from all over the world were encouraged to post new or unusual disease occurrences, and others were invited to provide insight or advice. ProMED has since grown into a large, effective international network with instantaneous reports of new or emerging diseases from even the remotest parts of the planet. It is the scientific community at its best.

The posting that day was a letter from the Australian chief veterinary officer to the director general of the Office International des Epizooties in Paris. In it, the veterinarian described the deaths of fourteen horses from an acute respiratory syndrome between September 7 and September 26, 1994. The horse trainer also died of a similar acute respiratory infection, on September 27. The agent was unknown.

The newly identified virus eventually took on the name of the suburb of Brisbane where the outbreak occurred—Hendra. A dozen horses, one man: one could say it was not something to lie awake at night worrying about.

In late 1998, also on ProMED, reports came out of Malaysia about an outbreak of Japanese encephalitis, caused by a virus related to West Nile virus and transmitted by mosquitoes. Since Japanese encephalitis is endemic in that part of the world, these reports were interesting but not terribly surprising. By December, eleven people had fallen ill and four had died; farms were fogged with insecticides, people were vaccinated, and the outbreak was declared over. By February 1999 there were twenty-five cases, with thirteen deaths; in mid-March, it was reported that ninety-eight people had fallen ill, forty-four of them fatally, within a three-day period. Thousands of homes and pig farms had been fogged with insecticides and thousands of people vaccinated with a Japanese encephalitis vaccine. Later the same month, there were reports that abattoir workers in Singapore had come down with encephalitis after slaughtering pigs from Malaysia. Japanese encephalitis is transmitted by mosquitoes. How could this be Japanese encephalitis? Was this, in fact, not Japanese encephalitis but a new disease?

Shortly afterward, the disease was being described as "Hendra encephalitis," and later, because it first appeared in the village of Sungai-Nipah, as Nipah virus encephalitis.

A new disease, characterized by fever and coughing followed by drowsiness and sometimes a coma, seemed to have come out of nowhere. It seemed to start in pigs and spread from there to dogs and people; older animals were more likely to become severely ill, with unsteady gait and frothing at the mouth. Scientists and investigators from around the world joined forces to investigate.

Reports from the Centers for Disease Control and Prevention in Atlanta sounded both excited and anxious. This virus had never been seen before. No one knew how it was transmitted or what it was capable of doing. Scientists wore gowns, gloves, and battery-operated respirators as they slogged their way through the pig farms at the center of the epidemic.

Even as the scientific investigation proceeded, the Malaysian army came in. More than a million pigs were slaughtered and buried. By the time the epidemic was over, in May 1999, 265 people from Perak, Negeri Sembilan, and Selangor states in Malaysia—mostly workers on pig farms—had fallen ill with encephalitis; more than a hundred died.

Where had the disease come from? Because pteropid bats (flying foxes) were suspected of being the main reservoirs of the related Australian Hendra virus, investigators pursued that avenue as one of several leads. Flying foxes (*Pteropus* spp.), which have a brain structure similar to that of primates and flying lemurs, are an interesting bunch. They are megabats, classified as megachiroptera to differentiate them (as if we couldn't tell) from microchiroptera, the microbats. Megabats have keen eyesight and roost in trees rather than in caves or houses. Some of the males sing in courtship. The females have single babies and nurse them at breasts. They eat fruit and nectar and are important for the survival and spread of flowering and fruiting plants in Africa, Asia, and Oceania.

Megabats carry around a variety of interesting viruses, including Hendra, Nipah, the viruses that caused severe acute respiratory syndrome (SARS), and Ebola and Marburg hemorrhagic fevers. Not only that, but a group of researchers from California State University have proposed that the Chamorro people of Guam, who have one of the world's highest rates of a fatal, progressive paralysis, amyotrophic lateral sclerosis, better known as ALS, or Lou Gehrig's disease, are being poisoned by a neurotoxin. This toxin, which comes the fruit of the palm-like cycad *Cycas micronesica*, is concentrated in, among other places, flying foxes, which the Chamorro cook up in coconut milk.

Megabats are important for the ecological sustainability of the planet. They are gregarious, and they are excellent social role models for children. They apparently taste pretty good, too, and are sold as food in many east Asian markets. And they are potentially deadly and not to be messed with. A lot like us, then.

But how would the virus get from fruit-eating bats to pigs and people working on pig farms? And why in 1998–99?

A plausible story that has emerged from the investigations brings together a complex set of interactions. Sadly, the story is both messy and increasingly common.

The El Niño–Southern Oscillation (ENSO) phenomenon is a huge natural cycle of oceanic and air currents across the southern Pacific. It was called El Niño by the Peruvians because it arrives just after Christmas, El Niño being the Spanish term for the Christ child. ENSO has been related to a wide variety of natural events, from the upwelling (and disappearance) of anchovies in Peru to monsoon rains and droughts in South and eastern Asia and all the way over to the east coast of Africa.

Scientists think that the ENSO cycles have been getting more frequent and more severe, probably as the result of human-induced climate change. The 1997–98 ENSO was the worst on record, resulting in a major drought through Southeast Asia. Even as the drought deepened, Indonesian forestry companies slashed through the forests of the area with wild abandon, and desperate Indonesian and Malaysian farmers set fires to clear land. That year, millions of acres burned out of control, and a haze of smoke covered the region, casting the landscape into shadow. Because the sun was blocked by the smoke, the forests and scrublands that were not directly destroyed by the fires suffered huge drops in a variety of crops, including many flowering and fruiting plants. This is where we get back to the fruit bats. With forests disappearing and fruiting and flowering plants deeply depressed in the smoky haze, the flying foxes were running out of options.

In the late 1980s, Malaysia (a Muslim country) had dramatically increased pig production to meet the needs of the Chinese in Southeast Asia, especially in Singapore, which was phasing out farming because it was running out of land. The Malaysians, being conscientious about land use efficiency, grew mango trees on their pig farms. In fact, mango production expanded at about the same rate as pig production in the 1980s and 1990s.

The Malaysians also let the pigs go into outside enclosures for fresh air. Guess what. The fruit bats found the fruit trees. They pooped into the open pig pens and dropped partially eaten fruits. The pigs, which will eat anything, ate everything; the virus came along for the ride. The viruses liked the pigs. Only a few pigs got sick, but the virus had a multiplicative heyday. The farmers picked up the virus from the pigs. Only a mass slaughter of pigs stopped the epidemic.

In several years following the epidemic, there were outbreaks of encephalitis, clinically appearing as fever, headaches, and "altered levels of consciousness," in Bangladesh and West Bengal State in India. In these countries, people who climbed date palms and drank raw palm juice were getting the disease. The palm juice was collected in open-topped clay pots. Fruit bats, feeding in the same trees, had apparently dropped half-eaten bits of fruit, as well as, possibly, feces, onto the pots. In this case the preventive measures were simpler and less traumatic than in Malaysia: put cloth covers on the pots.

SARS

At the end of May 2003, I was on a train and returning to Toronto from the Writers' Union of Canada annual general meeting in Ottawa. Outside the window, the countryside was greening into spring. Inside, it was all worry and fret. Several of my traveling companions wondered if they should be going to Toronto at all. A week after the World Health Organization had taken Toronto off an international travel advisory list for a newly identified disease called severe acute respiratory syndrome, a second epidemic wave was coughing its way across the city. More than two thousand people were in quarantine—which in Canada is a somewhat leaky concept, relying on goodwill and a sense of civic responsibility. Canada was unlikely to announce, the way the Chinese government did, that it would execute or jail for life anyone who broke quarantine.

In a democratic society, who out there might be spreading death and mayhem? Could we rely on a sense of public responsibility? Did my friends need to wear masks in the street? Would their lives be in danger? Remarkably, I reflected, despite my general cynicism about the self-centered consumerism of our culture, people did generally heed the call to quarantine themselves. When they broke quarantine, their activities seemed to be based on ignorance rather than bad will. There is more to admire in people, as Camus once said, than to despise.

Who would have thought that two deaths in Toronto could instill such fear? Sui-chu Kwan, a seventy-eight-year-old woman, died on March 5 of an apparent heart attack. A week later her forty-four-year-old son, Chi Kwai Tse, waited eighteen hours in an emergency room before dying of what was apparently tuberculosis. Yet, as two of the non-Chinese casualties of what has been called the twenty-first century's first pandemic, as indicators of both the consequences our past (in)actions and of our probable future, the deaths of Mrs. Kwan and her son have as great a significance as 9/11. Those of us who work near the health system were astounded at the chaos, infighting, backbiting, and heroism. Despite massive mobilization of doctors, nurses, epidemiologists, politicians, and weary volunteers, more than four hundred Canadians fell ill, and forty-four died.

Worldwide, eight thousand people got sick and more than eight hundred died. But the death toll is not really the story. The story is how awkwardly the most sophisticated, scientifically based medical systems in the world responded to what surely should have been a routine event: someone stricken with a potentially fatal infectious disease. The story is about a kind of cultural Alzheimer's disease and the cavalier satisfaction of the recently healthy.

The first cases of a kind of unusually severe and acute pneumonia had been reported from Guangdong Province in south China as early as November 2002. By February, cases were being reported in Vietnam. That month, Carlo Urbani, a physician and an officer of the World Health Organization, began documenting cases of this apparently new disease in a French hospital in Hanoi; by early March, he expressed concern that almost two dozen hospital workers had been infected. He called the new disease severe acute respiratory syndrome. "Syndrome" is the medical word used when you have a cluster of symptoms but you don't actually know if they reflect one disease, or, if they do, what that disease is.

By mid-March, cases had been reported from Hong Kong and Canada. High-tech laboratories around the world went into high gear to try to identify the agent, and the World Health Organization sent out a worldwide alert. Researchers had suggested that certain individuals might be "super-shedders"—that is, people who were spraying out extra-large numbers of viruses. Mrs. Kwan had returned to Toronto from a visit to Hong Kong, where she had stayed in the same hotel as a professor from China. The professor, unknown to himself, was a super-shedder.

WHO began to issue advisories warning travelers to avoid certain places if they could. By the third week of April, that list included not just cities in eastern Asia but also Toronto. By the time I was making my train trip to Toronto with my wary fellow writers, the travel advisory had been lifted, exhausted health workers were struggling to contain a new outburst of disease, and Dr. David Naylor, dean of the Faculty of Medicine at the University of Toronto, had agreed to lead a special advisory committee on SARS and public health.

Many of my colleagues have wondered how the Ontario health system had bungled things so badly and how the system might be fixed to prepare us for the next pandemic. How was it that Canadian researchers were able to sequence the genome of the offending virus more than a month before basic, low-tech public health measures could be applied to contain the disease?

Admittedly, gene sequencing is sexier than sharing data, developing clear lines of communication, and following hospital infection control procedures. I don't blame the gene sequencers. They were doing what they do best, and their work is ultimately important in tracing the origins of the disease. But, historically, diseases have not been controlled by gene sequencing; the most effective solutions are based on careful clinical observations and good old-fashioned health care, where "care" actually means care. Dr. Naylor's report on the Canadian response to the epidemic addressed many of those issues. Available online, it makes for some fascinating reading (at least for people interested in how the health care system functioned, or didn't, in times of duress).

The advisory committee that Dr. Naylor headed, set up by Carolyn Bennett, the astute federal minister of state for public health, among other things resulted in the establishment of the Public Health Agency of Canada, an agency that has since done much to identify possible emerging disease threats and to sort out strategies for dealing with them.

Whatever the problems were once the epidemic started, I was more interested in where this pandemic came from. In my view, people showing up at hospital doors with SARS or avian influenza represent failures of public health, no matter how slick, efficient, or triumphant the medical response. In the long run, it seemed to me, the important questions had to do with identifying how these diseases emerge in the first place. So where and how did SARS emerge?

Well, it seemed to come out of southern China in about 2002; that much was known. But why there? Why then?

In mid-March 2003, scientists working on the virus first suggested that it might be something related to measles and to animal diseases such as canine distemper and rinderpest in cattle, or at least in the same family, the paramyxoviruses. World health officials nodded their heads, and investigators went off looking for these viruses, which, in many cases, they found.

Other scientists then proposed a coronavirus, which under an electron miscroscope is said to have a corona, or crown. To me these viruses look like spheres with pins stuck into them, but I don't know a lot about crowns. Some types of coronaviruses cause the common cold; others cause respiratory disease in chickens (infectious bursal disease); still others are associated with diarrhea in dogs. The scientists called it SARS-coronavirus, or SARS-CoV. So the high-tech lab people had come through fast.

But what about the bigger questions about where the disease came from and hence how it might have been stopped or contained in the first place? Avian influenza had jumped from chickens to people in Hong Kong in 1997. Had SARS followed a similar path from animals to people?

Investigators familiar with the wide variety of animals farmed, caught, trapped, marketed, and eaten in south China, especially Guangdong Province, tested more than half a dozen types of animals from a market. They found evidence for the new virus in a raccoon dog and in several masked palm civets (*Paguma larvata*); although the latter are sometimes called civet cats, and they have a cat-like look, these fruit-eating, palm-dwelling animals are closer to mongooses.

Civets are gourmands of a sort. They love durian. Durian is a Southeast Asian fruit worth millions of dollars in trade and sales. When I lived in Java, a friend of mine who *liked* it declared it was like eating ice cream in an outhouse. The Indonesians wouldn't let people carry it on buses or airplanes because of its powerful odor but still swore by its wonderful taste.

Civets nose out a particular kind of Vietnamese coffee bean. The beans travel through the civet's digestive tract and, when they emerge, voila, they are *caphe cut chon,* or fox-dung coffee, which some people prize. From about the tenth century BC until recent times, civets have also been prized for their powerful musk, which was used to stabilize perfumes. Some (maybe a hundred a year) were imported to United States as pets; importing them into North America is now, as a result of their association with the SARS virus, forbidden. The Chinese and Vietnamese prefer to eat them.

In any case, once the finger was pointed at civets, thousands of them were slaughtered. Still, there were lingering doubts that civets were the natural reservoir and not simply part of the epidemic, which emerged from some other source. Investigators persisted. Apart from a situation in which a waitress and a customer in Guangzhou, China, picked up SARS in the winter of 2003–2004 from serving and eating civets near cages where the civets were kept before being eaten, the data were ambiguous. Could it be that civets were not the reservoirs at all, but were victims of the disease, or, at most, launch pads or amplifiers of the invading viruses, which came from elsewhere? Investigators could not find any widespread infection in either farmed or wild civets. Where else could a person look?

Bats also are found hanging around (unwillingly) in the markets of south China and Southeast Asia, where they are used for food and medicine. Given their history with Nipah and Hendra viruses, some scientists decided to check them out. All the bat species they tested had evidence of infection SARS-CoV-like viruses without being sick themselves. They were a perfect reservoir, silently infected, with no one watching them.

(10)

THE DARKNESS BLEEDS IN:

LASSA, EBOLA, AND MARBURG

*H*EMORRHAGIC FEVERS: the name says it all, and it conjures up many of our darkest fears. These diseases all, it seems, come out of the rain forests of Africa. They are described as "terrorizing" or "stalking" the human race. The agents are always "deadly," and they are "killers." They are reason enough for firebombing African villages and threatening to do the same to American cities, as in the movie *Outbreak*. They have names such as Lassa, Ebola, and Marburg. Marburg? Germany? Yes, and the strange thing is that if you are a virologist, used to looking at electron micrographs, you would say that Lassa was the one that doesn't belong. It's an arenavirus, you would say. The others are filoviruses; they look kind of stringy.

For non-virologists, what is more important is this: they all, more or less, start with malaise and aching muscles and then move on to high fever, coughing, diarrhea, pain everywhere, and, in the worst cases, bleeding all over, brain problems, shock, and death.

In 1969, a nurse in Lassa, North-Eastern State, Nigeria, came down with fever, aches, and pains—the unremarkable symptoms of serious tropical diseases such as malaria, or diseases of poverty such as typhoid fever. When she didn't get better after being treated locally, she was flown to a hospital in the Nigerian city of Jos. She died. One of the nurses who had taken care of her there also died. A third nurse, who had helped with the post-mortem of the first, became ill and was flown home to the United States in a commercial airliner. The Yale Arbovirus Unit isolated a virus from her blood and called it Lassa virus. A laboratory worker at the Yale laboratory fell ill, was treated with a transfusion of serum from the nurse, who was recovering and presumably had antibodies. The lab worker recovered. Five months later, another laboratory technician at the lab died of Lassa fever. No one knows how it happened.

The natural home of the Lassa fever virus is an African soft-furred rat, also called a multimammate rodent, *Mastomys natalensis*. *Mastomys* are at home in savanna woodlands common throughout parts of sub-Saharan western Africa. The rodents are sometimes described as pests and sometimes as food. I guess that depends on where they are found and how hungry you are.

Lassa fever virus belongs to a larger family of rodent lovers. Members of this family include Machupo virus (causing Bolivian hemorrhagic fever), Junin virus (Argentinian hemorrhagic fever), Guanarito virus (Venezuelan hemorrhagic fever), and lymphocytic choriomeningitis virus (found in Europe and North America and causing "flu-like" lymphocytic choriomeningitis disease, or LCM, and only rarely meningitis in people).

In the early 1970s, Lassa was considered a rare disease, which killed about half the people it infected, mostly in hospitals. But then, many diseases are considered serious when first discovered, simply because the most serious cases are the ones first reported. For a few years, small outbreaks with high death rates were reported from hospitals in Nigeria and Liberia. Then, investigators of a hospital outbreak in Sierra Leone reported that less than

10 percent of the people infected there picked it up in the hospital. The case-fatality rate was less than 5 percent.

Using this news as a starting point, an intrepid group of investigators from the Centers for Disease Control and Prevention in Atlanta, led by Karl Johnson and, later, Joseph McCormick, set out to describe the epidemiology and ecology of the disease in its natural setting. They found that the disease was endemic in much of western Africa. A few hundred thousand people a year may get infected, and 15 percent of them die with "multisystem" failure—which basically means that all their body organs shut down.

Occasionally, people still pick up Lassa fever virus in Africa and carry it home to other parts of the world. In 2004, a businessman returned to New Jersey after a five-month stay in Liberia. Toward the end of his visit to Africa, he developed fever, chills, sore throat, diarrhea, and back pain. Doctors in the hospital in Trenton, New Jersey, treated him with antimalarial drugs and antibiotics (for typhoid fever). He got worse and had trouble breathing. The doctors went down their list of possibilities and came up with yellow fever and Lassa fever as candidates. Both of these require expensive antiviral treatments. He died before they could start treatment. Since getting sick, he and/or his bodily fluids (blood) had come into contact with fellow airplane passengers, train passengers, family members, and laboratory workers. Nobody else, fortunately, got sick. But they could have.

In 1967, twenty-five laboratory personnel in Frankfurt and Marburg, Germany, and in Belgrade, Yugoslavia, fell acutely ill with high fevers, muscle and joint pain, vomiting, diarrhea, rashes, and bleeding, both internally and from the nose. Some of the people who took care of them also got sick. One spouse was infected through her husband's semen. Seven of the infected people died.

All of those originally infected were working with tissues and blood from African green monkeys (*Cercopithecus aethiops*) imported from Uganda. Cell lines derived from African green monkeys are used for vaccine research and various kinds of testing. For instance, the disease associated with the infamous *E. coli* 0157:H7, sometimes called hamburger disease, is also called verotoxin-producing *E. coli*. The actual disease is caused by a so-called verotoxin, which means that it kills African green monkey kidney cells in the laboratory. The original monkeys had not appeared to be ill, but there had been daily deaths among the monkeys in transit from Uganda, and experimentally inoculated monkeys of various sorts did become ill and die. Still, some of the African green monkeys experimentally infected did not get sick.

Almost a decade later, in 1976, dramatic epidemics of a hemorrhagic disease struck southern Sudan and northern Zaire. In the Sudan, about three hundred people got sick and more than half of them died; in Zaire (now the Democratic Republic of the Congo), about three hundred people got sick, and about 80 percent of them died. The virus that was isolated from the victims looked exactly like the Marburg virus, but it turned out to be something different. Doctors called it Ebola virus, after the Ebola River, one of the headwaters of the Congo (Zaire) River.

In the twenty years after that, only half a dozen incidents of Marburg virus disease were recorded, in Kenya, South Africa, and Zimbabwe, involving altogether a few dozen people, about a quarter of whom died. This changed abruptly in 1998, when an outbreak of Marburg disease started among "unofficial" gold mine workers in the Democratic Republic of the Congo; 149 people were struck with the disease and 123 of them died. Then, in 2004 and 2005, an outbreak of fever, vomiting, coughing, hemorrhaging, and diarrhea was reported from northern Angola. One hundred and twenty-four people got sick; three-quarters of them were children under five years. Of those who were sick, 117 died.

The disease seems to come out of nowhere but spreads among people who have very close contact with each other, either in hospitals or through burial practices. Then the disease disappears. Where does it come from? Where does it go back to? No one knows.

Initial suspicions fell on the monkeys as a reservoir. The monkeys in Marburg had been imported from an island in Lake Kyoga, that shallow, swampy lake near Mount Elgon, on the Kenya-Uganda border—the same (pleasant) area where our sleeping sickness work was done (see chapter 5). There were rumors that there had been a large number of monkey deaths in the wild colonies there, but these rumors were not corroborated.

A little more is known about the ecology and epidemiology of Ebola virus fever. Since the 1976 epidemics, scientists have determined that there are at least four different strains of the virus. The Maridi strain, which has struck in southern Sudan and northwest Uganda, kills from a third to two-thirds of its victims. The Zaire subtype, involved in attacks in Zaire, Gabon, the Democratic Republic of the Congo and the Republic of Congo, kills from 60 to 90 percent of its victims. The third African strain, from the Ivory Coast, is known to kill chimpanzees but not people. Another strain of Ebola, the Reston virus, was isolated from monkeys at a quarantine station in Reston, Virginia; the cynomolgus monkeys (and the virus) came from the Philippines, and, although it has been capable of killing the monkeys and instilling panic in the general public, this strain does not appear to cause serious disease in people.

The frequency of serious outbreaks of Ebola virus seems to be increasing in Africa, and there has been a concerted effort to find the natural reservoir for the disease. Scientists investigating five recent outbreaks of the Zaire strain in Gabon and the Republic of Congo found that the index cases (the sick people who start the epidemic) were people who handled dead gorillas, chimpanzees, and duikers. These animals are important sources of what is called bush meat, that is, wild-caught meat. The primates are particularly dangerous, because for a microbe, the jump from a monkey to a human being is more of a small step than a great leap.

People eat wild primates and other bush meat because they (the people) are poor and hungry and the animals are freely available to anyone with a gun. As people probe or are pushed deeper into new ecosystems in search of food, the bush meat trade has become a continuing potential source of new diseases, including, probably, several strains of the viruses that cause AIDS. The human epidemics of Ebola virus fever appear to have been preceded by, or associated with, deadly epidemics in animals, and biologists are afraid that Ebola may be devastating some wildlife populations in central Africa.

In all the Ebola outbreaks studied so far, once a person is infected, the epidemic is spread by close contact between the sick individual and his or her caregivers and through burial rites and the preparation of bodies for those burials. Controlling the spread of the disease thus requires culturally sensitive engagement with local people; caring for loved ones, and burial rites, are profoundly rooted in history and culture and are not changed through lecturing from medical experts. Often the very techniques that are so effective for treating disease (chain of command, control, reliance on technical expertise) are the least effective for promoting prevention and long-term health. To their credit, many medical organizations, including the World Health Organization, are discovering the value of anthropologists and of building local trust.

The reservoirs of both Ebola and Marburg viruses have remained elusive. If the wild primates are dying from the disease, they make a lousy natural home. Investigators have tried to narrow down the possibilities by studying the ecological situation and the geographic scope of the disease. Of the thousands of animals tested, the most promising candidates for reservoirs, as of late 2005, were several species of African fruit bats, which seem to be infected without becoming sick.

The good news is that these bats don't migrate beyond Africa and that if we can work together to establish sustainable communities in that troubled continent, to educate women and children and men, to build effective farming practices and create meaningful employment, the disease can be contained.

The bad news is that people move themselves and a wide range of species, legally and illegally, out of Africa every day. The animals are transported to become pets, to be used in research, or for food, or just because that's what humans do. In 2003, monkeypox (fortunately not a fatal disease in people) got into the United States when an animal distributor imported a variety of rodents from Ghana. These included species such as rope squirrels (*Funiscuirus* sp.), tree squirrels (*Heliosciurus* sp.), Gambian giant rats (*Cricetomys* sp.), brushtail porcupines (*Atherurus* sp.), dormice (*Graphiurus* sp.), and striped mice (*Hybomys* sp.). The animals were then shipped to pet stores across the country and housed in the same stores that sold prairie dogs, those pesky things that farmers like to shoot. Apparently, there is a market for these little beasties as pets; apparently, the market does not know that these animals act as vessels for microbes out to see and colonize the wide world.

It may be time to re-examine some of the things we "just do."

SPLASHING THROUGH RAT PISS:

LEPTOSPIRES AND HANTAVIRUSES

*S*WARMS OF little rodents and warm, wet weather are a
problem not just for the plague and Lyme disease but also
for another group, or clade, as some microbiologists refer to it, of
spirochetes, the leptospires. Leptospirosis, the disease, is caused
by more than 250 species of spirochetes and is the most common
zoonosis in the world.

In mid-June 1998, more than eight hundred triathletes lined
up on the shore of Lake Springfield, Illinois, for the sixteenth
annual Springfield Ironhorse Triathlon. These were healthy
young men and women, ready to swim 1.5 miles in the clean mid-
western lake, bike 45 miles across the flat landscape, and then
run another 10 miles. Swimming unseen alongside them in the
water were little schools of leptospiral bacteria, which insinuated their way undetected across the mucosal surfaces of the eyes,
mouths, noses, vaginas, and penises and into the bloodstreams of
these athletes.

For the next couple of weeks, the tiny speedster bacteria
dashed around the blood vessels until they got stuck in a variety
of small capillaries, especially in the kidneys, where they stirred
up trouble, causing local damage and bleeding. A week to two

weeks later, dozens of these prime young specimens were suffering from fever, chills, headache, muscle pain, diarrhea, and red eyes. Twenty-three were hospitalized. Nobody told them that rats or cows or some other animals had been peeing into the lake or that rats carry not only plague or hantaviruses but also, often chronically, in their kidneys, leptospires that they chronically piss out into the environment. Nobody told them that leptospires love to hang out in fresh water, damp soil, mud, and vegetation. Maybe they thought that the white-water rafters who picked up the same disease in Costa Rica in 1996 were somehow different. That was Central America, after all.

Given a few economically privileged adventurers complaining of muscle pains and fevers, one might be forgiven for not lifting this disease to the top of the global agenda. None of them, after all, came down with the most severe form of the disease, which results in kidney failure, bleeding from the lungs, and jaundice.

This severe form is called Weil's disease, not after the French mystic Simone Weil, although her passion for the poor and for God would suit those populations who suffer most from Weil's. Less interestingly, the disease was named after Adolf Weil, a nineteenth-century physician, who described it but didn't actually discover it. Japanese researchers early in the twentieth century discovered the spiral organisms with hooked ends in the kidneys of coal miners, among whom the disease was common, and also showed that rats were the primary carriers. Much of the early work was carried out in the warm, moist environments of South and eastern Asia.

A few queasy triathletes did not succeed in putting the disease very high up on the U.S. worry list. Most of the world, however, does not live in North America. Dairy farm workers in New Zealand get peed on by infected cows, and throughout the tropics millions of workers in rice fields, cane fields, or mines wade through, and occasionally accidentally imbibe, the pee of rats or other small mammals. Although rats are considered the chronic carriers (in their kidneys), dogs, cows, and pigs can also carry and shed leptospires. Livestock or dogs can be vaccinated, but the vaccine prevents disease; it doesn't prevent the organisms from snuggling up in the kidneys, and it doesn't prevent the little sportster spirochetes from shooting the yellow rapids out the urinary tract. Most of the time the organisms infect the kidneys, damage a few small blood vessels so that the blood leaks out, and cause a bit of fever but don't do anything more serious than that.

What is more worrisome—if you are looking for something to distract you from worrying about where the kids are tonight—is this: in 1995, after Hurricane Mitch flooded Nicaragua, two thousand people fell sick and more than a dozen died. They *did* bleed from the lungs. Between 1996 and 1998—just before and during a major ENSO event—there were serious outbreaks in Ecuador, Peru, and Brazil.

In 1996, in one hospital in Salvador, Brazil, several hundred people got the disease, of whom fifty died. The best predictors of whether patients would die were "altered mental states," "respiratory insufficiency" (that is, they couldn't breathe), and kidney failure. That same year, over just two months (February and March), fifteen hundred cases were reported in Rio de Janeiro. Not surprisingly the most important predictors of getting sick had to do with living in steep areas where there was poor sewage management, poor garbage collection, and no distribution of clean water. Studies in Peru found that living in slum conditions and not wearing shoes in the field put you at risk of getting sick. Go figure. It seems somewhat pointless to post an advisory, as the Centers for Disease Control and Prevention did for Lake Springfield, to stay away from the water.

Attending large recreational events and living in slums apparently are the two biggest predictors of where the disease is likely to hit. I suspect these two do not include the same people. And which activity do you suppose is likely to have more resources devoted to solving its problem?

Leptospirosis appears to be increasing in dogs in many parts of the world, probably, in part, because of global warming. Furthermore, there is shifting in the types of leptospirosis that are infecting animals. The strains vaccinated against are less likely to multiply and spill into the environment. As is happening with avian influenza, vaccination is inadvertently selecting for different strains. The vaccines don't cross-protect. The bacteria breed and evolve a lot faster than we and our much-vaunted biomedical technologies are capable of. And when sudden, heavy rainfalls occur as part of climate change, the rats piss and run (urinate and migrate, for the non-veterinarians who are reading this). Where they run to is where billions of people in the world now live—large urban slums.

While we are on the subject of problems associated with small rodents, it is worth mentioning hantaviruses. This family of viruses is spread from small, wild rodents to people when the animals' saliva, feces, and urine are aerosolized, and people breathe it in with dust. Not a pretty thought.

The Four Corners area of the southwestern United States is a Navajo Tribal Lands area on a high plateau where Utah, Colorado, New Mexico, and Arizona meet. In the spring of 1993, people began wandering into local medical centers with what at first appeared to be common flu-like symptoms: fever, muscle aches, coughing. The only trouble was that after the first day or so, the illness it didn't behave like the flu. Of the first dozen or so who showed up at the medical centers, about three-quarters died rapidly from respiratory failure. In the week after May 14, near Gallup, New Mexico, a young athlete, his fiancée, and four other people died. Over that summer, dozens more people came down with this new disease, and the case-fatality rate dropped, but not dramatically enough to make everyone relax.

The Centers for Disease Control and Prevention did what it does best. It mounted a concerted effort to isolate and identify the infectious agent, right down to its molecular structure. The people at CDC may sometimes be arrogant and bad at dealing with a lot of ecological and social determinants of disease, but they are *really* good at this lab stuff. They were able to identify a previously unidentified hantavirus, which was named, appropriately, *sin nombre* ("no-name"). The disease was called hantavirus pulmonary syndrome.

Since 1993, scientists have learned a lot about this family of viruses. In the early 1950s, during the Korean War, more than three thousand United Nations troops came down with a "new" disease that authorities called Korean hemorrhagic fever. No one really knew what was causing the acute fever, bleeding, and kidney failure; 10 to 15 percent of those affected died. That version of the disease is now called hemorrhagic fever with renal syndrome, which is somewhat more clinically (but somewhat less historically) informative. More than a hundred thousand people suffer from it every year in China alone. The actual virus wasn't identified until 1976, when Korean investigator Ho-Wang Lee isolated it and named it Hantaan virus, after a river in the demilitarized zone, where the disease is common. The medical diagnosis in the troops was made more than forty years after they got sick, based on stored serum samples and medical records. It is one of those cases that I use to justify not throwing out all those boxes of stuff that might be useful some day.

Variations on this disease, caused by a whole family of similar viruses, have been reported from places as distant from each other as Scandinavia and Manchuria, going back to the early part of the twentieth century. In Scandinavia, the disease seemed less serious than the Asian form and was called nephropathia endemica, which means it is a disease that is always around and affects the kidneys. Another form, similar to that in Asia, occurs in the

Balkans. Some investigators have suggested that viruses from the same family may contribute to chronic hypertension and kidney disease in the United States.

At about the time the 1993 outbreak was pumping adrenaline through the bodies of medical investigators, James LeDuc and several colleagues from the World Health Organization summarized much of what was known about hantaviruses to that point, suggesting that "they are very widely distributed and likely to be responsible for human disease in many parts of the world where they are not now recognized." Since that was written, an increasing number of cases and outbreaks have been "recognized" in North and South America, and a great variety of both viruses and rodent reservoirs have been identified. Researchers have also done detailed investigations into the lives of small rodents, their diseases, and human relationships to them. Apart from the Norway rat, which can carry the disease, other carriers include the deer mouse, white-footed mouse, bandicoot rat, meadow vole, reed vole, musk shrew, European common vole, yellow-neck mouse, small-eared pygmy rice rat, Mexican harvest mouse, cotton rat, prairie vole, California vole, vesper mouse, long-tailed pygmy rice rat, and Siberian lemming.

In "To A Mouse, on Turning Up Her Nest with the Plough," Robbie Burns lamented (as far as I can tell, struggling with my devil's tongue English understanding of the Scot's mind) disturbing the home of the little field mouse and the rupture with nature that her terror signified. "Wee, sleekit, cowrin, tim'rous beastie, / O, what a panic's in thy breastie!" he wrote to his "fellow-mortal" and "earth-born companion."

Had Burns known about hantavirus pulmonary syndrome, he might well have panicked himself—and our language and culture would be the poorer for it. Many cases in North America occur when people clean out cottages in the spring, disturbing nests and sending up clouds of mouse excretions. In Canada, Alberta has reported more than thirty cases since 1989, about a third of whom have died. The most recent outbreak, in 2005, involved four people near Edmonton, one of whom died. Although disturbing the nests of rodents explains individual cases, it doesn't usually explain outbreaks. In these instances, some combination of human behavior and ecological change is usually at work.

To understand these, we have to cast a wider net. In the several years before 1992, the Four Corners plateau was its usual semi-arid self. That year, as part of the El Niño-Southern Oscillation, heavy rains fell. These rains led to a big crop of piña nuts. A big crop of piña nuts meant a much better survival rate and population boom for field mice. The spring of 1993 was an especially mousy year on the high plateau. The *sin nombre* virus (like all the hantaviruses) circulates in the rodents without causing much damage. It goes to the kidneys and lungs, and the little rodents appear to shed the virus indefinitely. The extra rodents invaded the cabins and cottages. More excreta to clear out. More contact with people. More cases.

Later, as if anticipating the medical-scientific obsession with predictive planning and control, worried maybe that people will try to control the weather, Burns cautions that "The best-laid schemes o' mice an' men / Gang aft agley." In trying to control everything, we have to come face to face with ourselves.

If the message of hantavirus pulmonary syndrome for North Americans is that we should wear face masks while cleaning out the cottage and be especially careful after a mild, rainy winter and spring, the message from the larger picture of these rodent-borne diseases is more serious. How do humans come into contact with all these rodents? People are driven to clear marginal land, and they disturb the "cowrin" beasties. They crowd into slums, and the rodents come to live with them. Perhaps we are seeing more diseases like leptospirosis and hantavirus pulmonary syndrome because we are looking harder for them. But I suspect there is more to it, having to do with poverty, inequity, and reckless use of the planet whose care has been bequeathed to us.

If wealthy people can sometimes protect themselves from ills carried by rodents, I confess it gives me some small satisfaction to see how the subtle voices of nature manage to slip past our expensive and sophisticated technico-medical defenses and catch our notice. Rodent excreta in the cottage. Rodent piss in the lake. "We are in the air," they whisper. "We are in the water. You are us."

(12)

ALL THE RAGE

*I*N FRENCH, rabies is called *la rage*, which is appropriate. Rabies draws on seemingly inexhaustible wells of fear and anger. The reasons for this go to a deep human anxiety about some dark wildness at the heart of nature. The wild beast is out there, just waiting for us, and the images of slavering dogs and their wild cousins, the wolves, are the face of that beast. Of the 40,000 or so people who succumb annually to this terrifying disease, most are in the poor countries of the Southern Hemisphere, probably a quarter of them in India. In China, four epidemic waves, occurring at ten-year intervals from the mid-1950s on, killed at least 100,000 people. In the most severe of these, in the 1990s, more than 55,000 people are known to have died. Since the late 1990s, the number of human cases in China every year has increased dramatically; in 2004, more than 2,500 people succumbed. Most victims have been bitten by dogs. The statistics in China and India, the countries with the two highest death tolls, are not very accurate, however, since those who die are often poor people in slums or remote villages.

The story of rabies gets more complicated almost every day, certainly every decade. It used to be considered a disease of "mad dogs" that then bit people, and historically, that was mainly true. In much of the world, it still is. By the twenty-first millennium A D, other narratives about rabies had been constructed, based on a more complete scientific understanding.

After World War II, an epidemic of fox rabies swept out of the Soviet Union and westward across Europe. In the 1950s, fox rabies invaded southern Canada from the north, where it settled comfortably into the fox and skunk population.

Raccoon rabies was first recognized in Florida in the 1950s. From an initial small area, the disease spread north and west at about 25 miles per year. Then, in the 1970s, raccoon rabies was given a big boost; hunters from West Virginia decided they needed more raccoons to shoot and so brought several truck-loads of them north. At least one raccoon in the bunch had rabies. By the 1980s and 1990s, the raccoon rabies was speeding north through towns, cities, attics, and barns. By 1999, the rabid raccoons had reached the St. Lawrence River and were making their first crossings into Canada, just as Ontario had brought fox rabies under control through a wildlife vaccination program. There are two to three hundred raccoons per square mile in parts of southern Ontario: a disaster waiting to happen.

Rabies is kept alive by skunks in the Great Plains, coyotes in Texas, vampire bats in Latin America, and insectivorous bats just about everywhere. In the past decades, not only have scientists identified a much wider range of animals that harbor rabies than once was thought, but they have also identified different strains of virus. Some types of rabies virus are better adapted to raccoons, others to foxes, and still others to bats. In the mid-twentieth century, rabies was thought to be basically one disease, although a few oddball rabies-like viruses had been identified in Africa with names such as Oulou Fato (causing a non-fatal disease in dogs) and Duvenhage virus (which caused something that looked exactly like rabies but apparently wasn't). Fifty years later, the scientific literature was carrying reports on "rabies-like" lyssaviruses discovered in bats in Australia, Southeast Asia, Europe, and a variety of other unexpected places. The closer one looks, the more complex the picture seems and the less stable and homogeneous the virus appears.

The word "rabies" itself comes from the Sanskrit *rabhas*, 3000 BC, and means "to do violence." Chinese records from 555 BC use the same word for "mad dog" and the human disease hydrophobia. The Greek word *lyssa* is derived from a root meaning "violent"; according to Gerald Moss writing on mental disorder in antiquity (see Brothwell and Sandison, *Diseases in Antiquity*), *lyssa* originally seems to have meant "the rage that possesses the hero," but, in the *Iliad*, *lyssa* is connected with "dog," as in "mad dog."

So the connection between mad dogs and clinical rabies, often referred to as hydrophobia, is very old. Descriptions of rabies, connecting mental derangement, fear of water (hydrophobia), and the association with mad dogs go back to the twenty-third century BC, in Babylon. Three hundred and fifty years before Louis Pasteur, Girolamo Fracastoro, an Italian scholar, described both the disease and the means of transmission.

"Lyssaviruses" is the name now given to the group of viruses to which rabies virus belongs. Lyssaviruses are members of rhabdoviruses, which are rod shaped, with one end flattened and the other rounded, like a bullet. This may be an appropriate shape, given the seriousness of the disease.

The viruses, once insinuated through the skin into the muscle, multiply, find a nerve, and then float up the axon toward the brain, periodically pausing at junctions of nerve cells to reproduce. This trip to the brain may take anywhere from a few weeks to more than a year. Once in the brain, the viruses multiply again and then travel out the nerves to all the body's organs, including the salivary glands. With its brain commandeered and damaged by the viruses, the animal behaves in strange ways.

There are two main forms of the disease: furious rabies, in which the animal attacks unsuspecting victims; and dumb rabies, in which the animal mopes around and sinks into depression. An interesting study using game theory calculated that the best strategy for viruses to perpetuate themselves in animal populations would be to have variable incubation periods, variable symptoms, and variable social behaviors. It is pretty hard to learn which animals to avoid if they exhibit no consistent patterns. Natural selection (or an evil god) seems to have provided for just such a wild-card combination.

Although descriptions of the disease, and its connection with badly behaving dogs, have been around for a long time, describing this devilish disease clinically did nothing to make it go away or even to tame it. Historically, some people killed themselves when they were bitten by what they thought was a rabid dog, more terrified of the disease than of a possibly judgmental Creator. Other treatments have included holding people under water until they got better or drowned, a case of trying to treat the symptoms (fear of water) without getting at the cause, or feeding them various parts of chickens or dogs. No treatments, including the best technologies at our disposal today, are effective once the clinical signs set in.

Since the prehistoric human emigration from the gardens of our African and Middle Eastern Edens, dogs have been our most constant and faithful friends and companions. When we were hungry hunters, they guided us to prey. They have guided and guarded our sheep and cattle, sometimes paying for it with their lives. When we settled into agriculturally based settlements, they guarded our properties, barking at the approach of strangers. Our collective lives seem to have been a long march to the ultimate control of nature, and dogs have been a happy part of that march.

Control of nature has brought us many benefits. We grow genetically improved maize and coffee in neat, fertilized fields, accompanied by our tail-wagging canine friends, whom we have taught obedience. But nature has dark secrets. Just when we think we have control, it slips away. Volcanoes that seem to be asleep erupt in a grand, destructive passion. The dogs turn on us, snarling and biting and bringing death and madness; it is as if our own children were attacking us. Thus, when Louis Pasteur, in the last great scientific effort of his life, tackled rabies, he was facing the demons that always haunt us: the ones that say, what if all the things we think are normal and good suddenly turn on us?

Pasteur didn't need to stare down one of the most fearsome zoonotic diseases in history. He had figured out why beer, wine, and milk spoiled and how to prevent it: pasteurization. He had saved the French silk industry from death by a disease that ravaged the silkworms. He had, quite spectacularly, discovered and publicly demonstrated how to prevent anthrax.

In May 1882, at the farm town of Pouilly le Fort just south of Paris, before the watchful eyes of a skeptical media, Louis Pasteur injected fifty sheep with virulent (disease-causing) anthrax bacteria. Half the sheep had been vaccinated with an attenuated form of the bacteria he had grown in the laboratory; the other half had been left alone. The twenty-five that were vaccinated lived. Those who were not vaccinated died. This was public science at its best. Some estimates are that the vaccination of sheep and cattle that followed saved the French enough money to cover their war reparations to Prussia for having lost the 1870 Franco-Prussian War.

Having a vaccine is great, but it is not a panacea. When a disease occurs sporadically, or if people are very poor, vaccination isn't practiced, which gives the disease a chance to make periodic comebacks. Anthrax is still with us, partly as a bio-terrorist threat, but more importantly as a zoonosis. The spores last in the soil for a very long time. Outbreaks still occur in animals in parts of Canada and the United States (often associated with bison or cattle on the range), southern Europe, and parts of Africa and

Asia. Human cases continue to occur in India, Turkey, and several other countries. In the United States in 2006, a man who carried dried goat hides back from Côte d'Ivoire came down with anthrax.

It is thus no stretch to say that by 1885 Pasteur had given the world strong teeth, Happy Hours, French silk pajamas, and a vaccine for anthrax. What better legacy could a man leave the world?

He didn't need to turn his mind to rabies. But he did it. No one at the time knew about viruses. Scientists such as Robert Koch had barely started sorting out the relationships between the much larger bacteria and disease. But Pasteur had figured out that the brain and spinal cord were the tissues most affected in rabid animals and most able to cause disease if injected into new animals.

Taking spinal cord tissue from rabid dogs, he injected it into rabbits, which also became rabid. He then took spinal cord from the rabid rabbits and allowed it to dry. The longer it dried, the less potent was the tissue in producing rabies. Starting with the "weakest" tissue he had, he injected dogs with more and more potent disease-causing tissues until the dogs were completely resistant. But would the procedure work in people? Pasteur wasn't sure he was ready to try.

On July 6, 1885, a mother from Alsace brought her nine-year-old son to Pasteur. On July 4, the boy had been badly mauled by a rabid dog. He could hardly walk. The mother pleaded. Could Pasteur use his miracle cure? With some trepidation, he began the treatment with rabbit spinal cord that had been air-dried for fifteen days. Over the next ten days, the boy was injected (under the skin) with increasingly potent mixtures. The boy, Joseph Meister, lived. Then a shepherd came for treatment. Then hundreds more people, until, by the time I came along (much, much later!) everyone knew about the dreaded—and very effective—Pasteur treatment. Traveling by truck, bus, train and on foot through Turkey, Iran, Afghanistan, India, and Nepal in the 1960s, I knew to stay away from strangely acting dogs. But I also knew about the fourteen painful shots in the stomach, which could save my life.

All of this seems very far away from many of us today. By the 1970s, when I went through veterinary college, a pre-exposure vaccine had been grown in duck eggs, which, I would think, was good for rabbit lovers but something of a conundrum for duck lovers. One of my classmates fainted while being vaccinated— perhaps, as an animal lover, pondering this conundrum. Now effective pre-exposure vaccines are grown in human tissue culture (another ethical dilemma). There are also effective post-exposure vaccinations, which are designed to block the virus from entering the nerves from the bite wound. These new post-exposure treatments are considerably less traumatic than the Pasteur treatment; they are called post-exposure prophylaxis (PEP), which sounds almost cheerful, with sexual overtones.

It seems that we have faced one of our darkest fears and won. We have tamed nature. For most of the world, however, this is a mirage.

For many people in North America and Europe, it is hard to imagine the situations in Guatemala, China, and India, where mad dogs and hydrophobia are not just figures of speech. Yet Guatemala, where beauty meets grief, and happy Mayans meet war and rabies, is only a holiday flight away. The beautiful old Quiche Mayan city of Quetzaltenango ("Xela"), Guatemala's second-largest city, set in a high mountain valley, does not immediately inspire terror. In October and November of 2000, rabies reared its ugly head, and four people died horrible deaths, all bitten by dogs. The Ministry of Health initiated a program to destroy stray dogs, but it ran out of strychnine and ran into protests from animal rights organizations.

The other animal carrying rabies in Latin America is the so-called "common" vampire bat, *Desmodus rotundus*. The very mention of this animal raises hackles. Vampire bats and people shared the same New World tropical ecosystems for some ten thousand years, and stories of these blood-feeding bats and the disease they carried have been part of some of the most ancient cultures in tropical America. However uneasy this relationship must have been, it was thrown way off kilter when the Europeans arrived with their cattle—blood for everyone! In the twentieth century, the main argument against vampire bats was not so much that they attacked people (which they occasionally did) but that they caused economic losses to cattle, both through causing paralytic rabies and from the effects of drinking blood.

Bats go back at least 50 million years. They are among the earliest mammals, and were here well before humanity stumbled on to the scene. They probably (mostly) came out of Laurasia, one of the two giant continents (the other being Gondwana) into which Pangaea, the original mother of all continents, split about 250 million years ago. Laurasia later fragmented into North America, Asia, and Europe.

Globally, there are about eleven hundred species of bats—20 to 25 percent of all mammals. In Latin America, there are nearly 250 species of bats; more than half of all mammals there are bats. Of the Latin American bats, about 70 percent eat insects, some of them up to five hundred insects an hour, which would be reason enough to protect them. But they may be just as important for flowering and fruiting plants, for pollination and seed dispersal. The list of plants that rely on bat pollination and spread in the wild includes everything from bananas and avocados to dates, figs, peaches, mangoes, tequila, and durian, although the last of these is, in my books, a somewhat dubious distinction.

Some bat pollinators can be considered "keystone" species: if they are eliminated, a cascade of extinctions could devastate the ecosystems in which they live. Fewer than one in a thousand, from three species, are vampires. When people first responded to vampire bat rabies, however, they did not know these things. They did not want to know. Whatever the motivation, the responses reflected the old, deep fear and rage and ranged from dynamiting, burning, poisoning, and gassing caves to leaving out poisoned bananas. Bananas for blood feeders? Clearly, the bats killed were not all vampires.

In the 1970s and 1980s, more targeted campaigns were mounted to vaccinate cattle or smear anticoagulants on them for the bats to pick up and then share with each other during grooming. In the 1990s, new patterns emerged. In some rural areas, when pigs and cattle rapidly disappeared (as many farms disappeared and livestock rearing was consolidated to respond to free trade "imperatives"), the bats looked for new sources of food and found people. In other cases, when people moved into wilderness areas—as in mining camps in the Amazon—and the bats' usual wildlife sources of food disappeared, they again looked to the delicate-skinned gourmet food—people.

Thanks largely to the works of scientific humanists like Pasteur, this dark, uncontrollable wildness at the heart of nature seems far away for many people in North America and Europe. In these places (with the exception of the Russian Federation), almost all the rabies reported is from wildlife (foxes, skunks, raccoons, mongooses, bats) and only in a few cases from domestic animals such as cats, dogs, or cattle. Human cases are rare in the United States and Canada, and for an increasing number of them, either we don't know how people got it, or the route of exposure was unusual.

Most years, no one gets rabies in Canada, the United States, or Europe. For the United States, 2004 was an exceptional year: four people died after receiving organ transplants from an infected donor. Two others were bitten by rabid dogs while outside the United States, and one person was infected from a bat but (unusually and perhaps miraculously) survived without having received vaccination ahead of time. When people do succumb, often weeks to months after exposure, it is indeed a terrible way to die. In Canada, the last case was in a boy from Quebec, in 2000. He was probably bitten by a rabid bat in the cabin where he had slept with his brother, although he was not aware of being bitten. His disease started with a fever and a pain in his arm on September 28 and ended on October 6 with hydrophobia, convulsions, salivation, and asphyxia.

One can understand why there has been a concerted effort in many parts of the world to eradicate the disease. I can even almost understand why, in Alberta in the early 1950s, the government started an all-out war that left in its wake the bodies of about 50,000 red foxes, 35,000 coyotes, 4,200 wolves, 7,500 lynx, 1,850 bears, 500 skunks, and 164 cougars. If it was not an act of science, its ferocity betrayed a passion that deserves, I think, respect.

In the late 1980s, Ontario started one of the biggest public health programs directed at rabies in the world. Many physicians and public health workers will be surprised to hear this information, because they have the mistaken notion that public health has something to do with the delivery of medical care. This supposition is only rarely true. When I began working as a veterinarian in Ontario, in the 1980s, there were fifteen hundred to three thousand cases of rabies per year in the province. This was one of the highest reported rates of any jurisdiction in the Western Hemisphere. I hasten to add that, unlike the situation in China, these were *non-human* animal cases.

Shortly after I arrived in Ontario, I visited a dairy farm to check on a cow that was "off her feed." She was a pretty normal-looking black-and-white Holstein. She just wouldn't eat, and she was a little wobbly in the hind end. In most places in the world, one might think of some physical injury or indigestion or perhaps a toxin. Then I had to remind myself that this was not just anywhere in the world. This was Ontario in the 1980s. If an animal acts strangely, think rabies. That is indeed what she had. It was also in this rabid context that, in August 1986, a woman delivered four cute puppies to a humane shelter in a Canadian city. What she did not tell the people at the shelter was that the pups, along with their mother, had been in contact with a fox on the farm where they lived. Nor did she tell them what her veterinarian had told her five days before, that all the dogs should be destroyed or quarantined.

The day they arrived at the shelter, two of the pups were taken to a nursing home as part of a visitation program. Over the next twenty-four hours, all four pups were adopted.

Over the next week, one of the puppies had diarrhea and vomiting and then died. A second also got sick and died. Although neither puppy was afflicted with a great rush of biting madness, both, it turned out, had rabies. A total of 139 people were required to have PEP. This disproportion between the event (exposure to one animal) and the post-exposure vaccination numbers is fairly common; 665 people needed PEP after exposure to a rabid kitten in New Hampshire in 1994, and 400 people were treated after a goat at a county fair in New York came down with rabies in 1996.

No one at the nursing home or shelter actually got rabies, whether because of luck or good management or PEP we can never be sure. The mother dog remained healthy through all these events. One of the local physicians, drawing on the deep fear I alluded to earlier, pontificated that this story showed why animals should not be allowed in nursing homes. But that is a simplistic focus on disease and ignores health completely. The appropriate lesson is that all relationships carry benefits and risks and that understanding can reduce but not remove risks. Andrea Ellis of Health Canada and I developed a little booklet,

Good for Your Animals, Good for You, which sets out rules for people who want to use animals in schools and nursing homes. The rules relevant to rabies are simple; wild animals that are friendly to people should be assumed to be sick until proved otherwise, and animals of unknown origin should never be put into contact with people until they (the animals!) have been properly vaccinated and observed for a couple of weeks.

But risk reduction for disease is ultimately not just a personal act. It is also a function of social programs. If the amount of rabies in the populations that surround us can be reduced, then the probability that people will come into contact with it will also be reduced, regardless of their behavior. If that can be done, we don't need to fear a descent into a hell of madness every time someone gets bitten.

Although most of the cases in Ontario in the 1980s were in wildlife, public health officials and physicians had to investigate 15,000 to 25,000 animal-human encounters every year, simply because the level of suspicion remained high. Because rabies was so common in animals, every animal bite could bring the deadly disease. Some farsighted biologists decided that the problem should be addressed at its source. Most of those wildlife cases, they discovered, could be traced back to the way the virus circulated in foxes. If the scientists could control fox rabies, they might be able to get a handle on the whole situation. Killing the animals, they realized, could well cause an even bigger epidemic as new, young (and sometimes rabid) foxes moved from the surrounding areas into the vacated territories and fought with each other.

The vaccination program was based on previous experience with vaccinating foxes in Europe, a series of astute field observations of fox behavior in Ontario, very clever mathematical models, and the hard work of some long-suffering wildlife biologists. They calculated that vaccinating about 70 percent of the foxes would bring the epidemic under control. The vaccine was delivered from airplanes, and by hand, in the form of edible baits. The baits are labeled "Do Not Eat," on the sometimes questionable assumption that people are more likely to read and obey such a warning than foxes. This taming of nature has been (if I may say so) wildly successful. The number of cases had dropped to fewer than one hundred per year by the new millennium.

Now, in North America, attention has focused on rabid raccoons, which have spread all through the eastern seaboard and are eyeing the land of better health care across the river at Niagara Falls, Canada, and on bats, since it is from them—or increasingly, from "unknown" exposures, which may or may not be bats or aerosolized bat excretions—that people are getting the disease. The second-to-last case in Canada was from a bat in northern Alberta; the last case, from a bat in Quebec. Still, globally, dog-related rabies accounts for 90 percent of all cases in people, and dogs kill lots more people than bats even when the pooches don't have rabies.

There are some effective responses to this global situation. Dog-population-control programs and vaccines, for instance, could bring rabies under control throughout the world pretty quickly. Louis Pasteur and his intellectual descendants would say, with very good reason, that we can experiment and think our way out of our fears. Pasteur urged his fellow citizens to worship in the sacred temples of scientific laboratories. He was convinced that in so doing, humanity would learn not just to conquer disease but also to turn away from fanaticism and barbarism and to find wealth, well-being, and harmony with nature.

Given Pasteur's lofty ideals, the death of one of his most celebrated patients was thus doubly tragic. In 1940, Joseph Meister, the man whose life Pasteur had saved with his vaccine, was serving as gatekeeper to the Pasteur Institute in Paris, when the German invaders—who, like their Soviet partners, pursued an ideologically driven, supposedly dispassionate science—

demanded that he open Pasteur's crypt. Rather than opening the crypt to the barbarians and thus desecrating the grave of the man who had saved, and given pleasure to, so many lives, Meister committed suicide.

Pasteur was a consummate scientist of his time. He brought the world into his laboratory, and then took the results back out to the world. He did not do his work in some secretive corporate or government laboratory, trying to make money, save face, or make a name for himself. He worked in the open and thus open to challenge. The network of scientific institutes he founded, beginning with the second Pasteur Institute in Saigon (now Ho Chi Minh City) in 1891, spans the globe.

But not all of humanity worships in the laboratory; many are kept out by language and money and a scientific culture of disciplinary obfuscation and exclusion. Vaccines are useless unless they are distributed and administered. Doing these things requires something approaching a sense of human solidarity and international justice. As we have seen with avian influenza, these instincts seem—at least at the governmental, political, bureaucratic level—to be in short supply. Furthermore, some of the solutions do not lie in the laboratory at all but in a deeper understanding of ecology and in human behavior. They require a new, more difficult kind of science.

Today, those of us who are scientists face the challenge of taking our work into the world, out of our very fine and expensive laboratories (knowing, thanks to Pasteur, that they are there to back us up). We need to ask questions that laboratory-based science cannot answer, to stand in the midst of the jungles and the farms and to begin asking the hard questions: not, how do we kill vampire bats or poison dogs or raise more cattle, but how do we nurture a convivial and complex and just world? Can we minimize infections and improve our food supply by how we design our living spaces? Can we control the residual diseases through

vaccines? Are vaccines, if they exist, widely available? Is ecological knowledge respected and pursued with the same energy that
new drugs and money-making technologies are invented? Do
we have rituals and songs and stories for dealing with inevitable
tragedy? The way we answer questions such as those will define
the quality of our science and of our humanity.

With All Our Most Constant Companions

. . .

DISEASES PEOPLE GET *from* ANIMALS

with WHOM WE HAVE MOST CLOSELY

SHARED OUR LIVES (PETS *and* LIVESTOCK)

. . .

(13)

ABORTION IN THE SANDBOX

AND OTHER PET PROBLEMS

Ironically, as the forerunner of animal domestication, pet-keeping led us into our present, destructive phase of history. Perhaps, by making us more aware of our biological affinities with animals and the natural world, it will help to lead us out again.

JAMES SERPELL, *In the Company of Animals*

THROUGHOUT THIS book, cats and dogs and other pets make several less-than-grand entrances, usually having to do with the quality and quantity of fecal matter they produce or with birthing fluids and materials or with their fleas. Given what is now known about the microbial world that surrounds us, are these companion animals nature's Trojan horses? Why do we bring them into our homes? (Why, indeed, my farm-born friends ask.) Are they bringing all manner of parasites, bacteria, and viruses into our homes? No doubt. I have friends who would say that all such animals belong in the barn or outside somewhere. Certainly a dog can do just fine sleeping in the straw, and cats can live on mice in the barn. We delude ourselves if we think they *need* the decadence of our houses. Still—even being a practical-minded Mennonite of agricultural heritage—I keep my cats in the house. What is going on here?

When I wrestle with my cats on the floor, rolling over and over, finishing with a good strong bite or an exuberant scratch from a feline, some self-obsesséd modern-day psychological snake-oil salesperson might say that I am getting in touch with my inner child. My literary friends might draw other inferences, something about genre blending, based on the cats' names: Gabe (the lionesque Gabriel García Márquez namesake) and Lenny (the sleek, all-black Leonard Cohen namesake).

Researcher James Serpell suggests that dogs and cats can express affection to their owners, but they cannot, verbally in any case, lie to them or criticize them. It seems that pets combine the benefits of human relationship with few of the threats. Anyone who has held a door open for an indecisive cat on a cold day, however, or had a dog chew up underwear, knows that human-animal interactions can be as annoying and frustrating as many human-human ones. And I have seen enough devious dogs to know that all this pets-are-wonderful stuff needs to be taken with a grain of salt.

So why, on a tight budget, when millions of children are starving in the world and environmental causes need all the financial aid they can get, do I fritter away money and energy by keeping these little beasts in the house? Are the cats ersatz therapists, or am I perhaps only toying with a substitute for the satellite dish I don't have? Do I harbor delusions of upper-class grandeur? Are cats my version of the ghetto Cadillac?

Keeping pets is a worldwide phenomenon not restricted to modern times or Western society. In 1978, a twelve-thousand-year-old tomb was unearthed in northern Israel that contained the remains of a human being and a dog. The dead person's hand was arranged to rest on the dog's shoulder. Native Fijians of a few centuries ago made pets of fruit bats, lizards, and parrots; Samoans were fond of pigeons and eels, and Hawaiian women were known to suckle puppies. Australian Aborigines kept dingoes, the Semang Negritos of Malaysia kept pigs and monkeys, and the Navajo Indians of North America shared their homes with cats. The upper classes of ancient Egypt, I'm told, revered dogs, cats, and various other animals. But then their priests also revered onions, so we might be somewhat skeptical of claims to exalted status in Egypt.

Apart from the eighteenth-century Ch'ing dynasty, when imperial Pekingese or lion dogs were suckled at the breasts of human wet nurses and attended by a retinue of palace eunuchs, pet keeping—until the recent upsurge in its urban, mall-based economy—does not appear to have taken a strong hold in China, and dogs there were more likely to be quaffed than be adorned with a coiffure. Pet culture is also relatively new in Europe. During the sixteenth, seventeenth, and eighteenth centuries, when Europeans viciously brutalized each other with religious zeal, it is not surprising that they had little empathy for other species and scoffed at New World aboriginal people who kept company with various raccoons, monkeys, peccaries, tapirs, wolves, bears, and the like.

People keep companion animals because they are seen to be useful or because they are demonstrably not useful. Muslim tribesmen in Sumatra still keep, and value, dogs for hunting pigs, both unclean animals. The dogs are happy because they get to eat the pigs, and the people are happy because they get to bend religious taboos without qualms. There are dogs for the deaf and for the blind and horses for the lame. Or an animal may be kept as an outlet for nurturing, care-giving behavior in a society that in the workplace assigns economics as the ultimate arbiter of what is good. In this respect, keeping a pet may be an act of rebellion against those utilitarian social values.

The therapeutic effects of pets have been much talked about and sometimes studied. The most commonly cited scientific study of the beneficial effects of pets is that reported by Erika

Friedmann and her associates in 1980; people who owned pets were more likely to survive a year after discharge from a coronary care unit than patients without pets. Other studies have shown demonstrable effects of pets in lowering blood pressure, improving morale, and facilitating social interaction. Nevertheless, the most influential and repeated stories of the physical and emotional benefits of pets are just that: stories. From a scientific point of view, they provide support for the greatest medical discovery of the twentieth century: the placebo effect, the ability of humans to heal themselves. The fact that pets can facilitate this process is not something to be taken lightly and would be reason enough to use pets in therapy.

In the 1990s, our research group, led by the epidemiologist Parminder Raina, studied the relationship of pets to health and health care costs in people over sixty-five. Raina found that, for people with good human social-support networks, pets had minimal effects. For those who lacked social-support groups (an enlarging population among the aged), pets provided an important buffer in times of crisis: the less human support they had, the stronger the positive effects of the pets in improving their mental and physical health. So, pets are more than just therapy, but they are not an unmitigated good. In some groups of people—those who actually don't like animals or are poor or overworked—pets can actually decrease health and morale.

I am currently working with another team to determine if dogs that visit hospitals as part of special visitation programs bring in possible zoonotic agents or carry them from patient to patient or take them out of the hospital into the community. Although most hospitals in North America have some sort of pet-visitation programs, these risks, and how to manage them, have only rarely been studied.

As a child, I used to visit my cousins on the farm during the summer and enjoy scaring the chickens and having my oldest cousin try to squirt milk from a cow's teat into my mouth. One summer, when I went home, I found that I had raised, reddish, circular marks on my arm. The doctor called them ringworm, which is not a worm at all, but a fungal infection of the skin and hair follicles common in many animals. As a veterinarian, I used to treat it in cows by using a good scrub brush, sunlight, and fluo-ride-containing toothpaste, which seemed to work as well as anything more "advanced" in my toolbox.

Fungal skin infections are among the most benign things we can pick up from animals. Most of these zoonoses go from other animals to people, but a few travel from people to other animals, and some can move in both directions. The 100 million or more dogs and cats in North America "threaten" us with at least thirty diseases. Even apparently innocent birds can fluff the air with intestinal bacteria and psittacosis (parrot fever) as well as with song. Pet turtles are notorious for spreading *Salmonella*, though I must confess that the turtle of my youth, Nikita, named after the Soviet leader Khrushchev, never gave me anything worse than a desire to escape from plastic dishes and leap daringly from table tops. This he did by his daring example, which finally succeeded in his escape from my attempts to domesticate him.

The good news is that in industrialized countries, except for bites and allergies, pets are rarely identified as culprits in making us sick. Even more rarely do they give us serious illnesses, despite thousands of intimate contact hours between them and humans. The most common zoonoses show up in people as general "flu-like" sickness (transient fever, headaches and muscle aches), skin problems, stomach problems, and bites or scratches. A few, like rabies, can kill you. And some are more than passing strange.

"Could Schizophrenia Be a Viral Zoonosis Transmitted from House Cats?" This is the title of a 1995 article published by two respectable scientists in the *Schizophrenia Bulletin*. The logic behind this idea was half-baked, but the hypothesis was intriguing. Although I might joke (in the privacy of my home, where after a few drinks I am known to use certain language that in public would invite a stoning) that my cats drive me crazy, it seemed farfetched to associate them with a serious psychiatric disorder.

If that earlier suggestion was open-ended and menacingly vague, a study reported in 2005, in *The Proceedings of the Royal Society*, asked a much more specific question. Could a parasite, in particular the cat-associated tiny parasite *Toxoplasma gondii*, be the causative agent of human affective disorders? The answer was stunning. J.P. Webster and a team of British and American researchers reported that rats infected with the parasite developed a suicidal attraction to cats. Furthermore, the researchers found that two antipsychotic drugs used to treat (among other afflictions) schizophrenia, as well as drugs that treated the infection itself, were capable of altering this rat behavior.

Many parasites have a definitive host, in which they reproduce sexually, and an intermediate host, in which they may undergo some development but don't sexually reproduce. *Toxoplasma gondii* makes its definitive host home in members of the cat family. That's where, in the mucoid comfort of the intestinal walls, the parasites have sex and make babies (cysts), which then move on, into the world at large, to make their homes elsewhere, in rodents, pigs, sheep, people, or whatever other animal happens to eat them. They always return to members of the cat family to have sex.

In kittens, *Toxoplasma* causes a transient diarrhea when they are first exposed to it, usually by eating infected mice. This lasts only a couple of weeks and seems to be the only time cats can pass the disease on to others. Hence we sometimes hear the admonition not to allow cats to hunt freely, lest they pick up the infection. I am considerably more concerned about the alarming negative impact on ground-nesting birds by millions of feral cats in the countryside than I am about transient diarrhea in kittens. But there is much more to it than this.

Having flooped their way out of the kitten's bum into the wider world, the little parasite cysts may, in a period of a few days to weeks (depending on temperature and moisture), develop into a stage where they can infect any warm-blooded animals, including people. Cockroaches can carry the cysts around in their guts for several weeks after feeding on cat feces; if they got sick, one might suggest that this is a fate that is well-deserved. They seem, however, just to carry the cysts from place to place, like the workhorses of the microbial world that they are.

Once inside the non-cat species, they slip out of their cysts with a little help from digestive enzymes, change into crescent shapes, and look for white blood cells called macrophages, which are supposed to eat bad invaders. The *Toxoplasma* parasite penetrates the cell and hangs out in the back seat of the cell-car, reproducing asexually as it is spread throughout the body, eventually settling into cysts in various tissues. There they await consumption by a member of the cat family. Well, they don't just wait. In many species, infection with *Toxoplasma* parasites results in abortion, stillbirth, and neonatal death; rats and cats can get reinfected by eating the dead fetuses. If the parasites are in a rat, they change the rat behavior. The rat-cat relationships described by Webster and his colleagues seem to have been an elegant co-evolution between the parasite, its intermediate host, and its definitive host. I don't know of any evidence that human attraction to cats is the result of a brain infection with *Toxoplasma*, although the world is a wondrous strange place, and I would not discount such a phenomenon.

Different forms of the parasite were described in Java sparrows (in 1900), gundis and rabbits (1908), and a whack of other species before researchers figured out that all the parasites they were looking at under the microscope were the same *Toxoplasma*.

It wasn't until the 1970s that scientists discovered the trysting, let's-have-sex-until-we-drop hideouts for *Toxoplasma*: cats. *Toxoplasma gondii* are now classified as members of a phylum called Apicomplexa, which also includes dinoflagellates, tiny non-plant/non-animal living things that thrive in the damaged coral reefs and can cause serious food poisoning, but that's another story.

Toxoplasma have inside them tiny organelles, called plastids, which resemble chloroplasts, those nano-biotech machines in plant cells that enable them to use sunlight to produce bio-energy and that are probably derived from an earlier, free-living ancestor that moved in and decided to stay. In a similar fashion, *Toxoplasma* today move into warm-blooded vertebrates of all kinds and stay there for life. The genus itself goes back some ten million years, making them somewhat older than us. Apparently there are three genetic lineages (or clones) today, which can be traced back to two parents about ten thousand years ago. They are, one might say, more numerous than the grains of sand on the beach. What the Creator promised to Abraham, he clearly promised to the original *Toxoplasma* ten times over. So we humans—ourselves a community of microbes—are parasitized, the parasites having been parasitized. A more positive spin is to say that we have learned that we function best as living beings when we recognize our interdependence and co-operate.

In people (and other animals), the parasite goes through the gut and crosses into the bloodstream, where it heads for the delectable tissues of the muscles, eyes, and brain. In one of its forms, it has a round bottom and a cone-shaped nose (a conoid), which can rotate, tilt, extend, and retract. Once in the lymph and blood, it gets around by gliding, undulating, and rotating, using its nose to find and penetrate host cells. The parasites are a quiet lot of immigrants. Most people who are infected aren't even aware of that infection. Most of those who become clinically ill might mistake the symptoms for mononucleosis: headache, fatigue, low-grade fever, and swollen lymph nodes. Some people get eye infections (chorioretinitis), which can result in weird visual effects.

Traditionally, doctors have worried most about toxoplasmosis in pregnant women. The women themselves just get the flu-like syndrome. It's the babies who suffer. Almost half the women who are infected during pregnancy either lose the babies (neonatal death or abortion) or give birth to congenitally infected infants. Babies can be born with a whole range of diseases from eye infections to pneumonia, jaundice, fevers, rashes, and severe neurological problems requiring lifelong care.

If a woman is infected before she gets pregnant, the parasites may cause a mild illness and are then kept out of the bloodstream by the mother's antibodies. In this case, the fetuses don't get infected. In other words, the babies of women who have had infection are safe, protected by the antibodies in the bloodstream; the babies of women who have no evidence of prior infection are in danger. The parasite can get in and go straight to the fetus.

As late as the 1980s, some experts recommended that we should arrange for all children to get infected. They would get a bit of flu. They would get over it. And the girls wouldn't have to worry about picking it up during pregnancy. The other options are expensive, and few publicly funded health care programs have shown any eagerness to promote them. Some countries, such as France, screen all pregnant women and warn those who don't have antibodies to keep especially clean and report any illnesses. They can then treat new infections as they come up. Other countries do this only on a voluntary basis, since running tests on everyone is expensive, and there is always the danger of a false positive test, which would cause the prospective mother to drop her guard.

The recommendation to infect the kids was all very well until AIDS, organ transplants, and immune-suppressing cancer treatments came along. Suddenly, in the 1990s, physicians were reporting that up to 40 percent of AIDS patients were coming down with severe encephalitis caused by *Toxoplasma*. What was happening? Were these new infections? Should people who are immuno-compromised avoid cats?

It turns out that no, people with AIDS, pregnant women, and people undergoing cancer treatments do not need to avoid cats, although doctors who are doing organ transplants should check to make sure they aren't passing on parasites hiding in the organs. The appearances of these serious brain infections in people with AIDS were almost entirely all the reactivation of old infections. In just about every country in the world, a third to half the population has had an infection with *Toxoplasma* by adulthood. The tiny cysts wait quietly around in the tissues, minding their own business, keeping out of the way of antibodies circulating in the bloodstream, but they are by no means dead. As soon as these community police disappear, the parasites come out and celebrate.

It is true that people can get infected by inadvertently eating kitten poop that has been sitting out for several days, although no one gets infected from eating *fresh* feces. The *Toxoplasma* oocysts need at least a couple of days to get ready for their next great adventure. It is only then, after a few days, that people can get infected. Thus, there was a lot of concern in the 1980s about contaminated playgrounds and sandboxes, which kittens were using as litter boxes. That was when I built the hinged wooden cover for the sandbox in our backyard. But the problem is more widespread than urban playgrounds and household cats. Who plays in a sandbox anymore anyway? Everybody's kid's got a handheld electronic telephone–game player–TV. Sandboxes are for, well, cats.

Cats in the countryside not only kill mice, which seems okay, and birds, which seems not to be, but also use grain bins as litter boxes. Who can blame them? Grain is such a comfy litter. Up to half of all North Americans are thought to become infected at some point, from a variety of sources. Many of us apparently get infected when we eat undercooked meat from animals that have eaten grain used by farm cats as a litter box. Although pigs have low rates of infection, we eat a lot of pork, so that seems to be an important source of exposure.

In Canada and the United States, we don't eat a lot of sheep, but sheep are raised under natural conditions, which makes not only the sheep happy but also the mice, cats, and parasites. In a study I did of Ontario sheep farms in the late 1980s, I found that almost all of them were infected. Among the factors that determined how common the infection was in the flock were access to flowing water and the number of kitten litters born on the farm every year: more kittens means more infection. At the time of the study, I wasn't quite sure what to do with the flowing water bit. Only one outbreak of water-borne toxoplasmosis had ever been reported, in American troops who drank from a jungle stream in Panama; they came down with fever, chills, and swollen lymph glands.

Then came 1995. Dr. Andrew Burnett was an ophthalmologist in Victoria, British Columbia. According to a report by Anne Mullens in the *Canadian Medical Association Journal*, in January 1995 Burnett saw a forty-nine-year-old man with floaters in one eye and complaints of hazy vision. Apart from an acute infection of the retina, he seemed healthy. Although the clinical disease is rarely diagnosed in British Columbia, Burnett suspected toxoplasmosis, which Raj Gill of the B.C. Centre for Disease Control laboratory in Vancouver confirmed. Over the next few months, Burnett and a fellow ophthalmologist, Stan Short, saw seven other cases with the same diagnosis. Gill, who was doing all the serum testing for *Toxoplasma* for the province, reported a sharp increase in positive results to Judy Isaac-Renton, a medical microbiologist at the lab.

What they were seeing, and what at the time they didn't know they were seeing, was the largest reported outbreak of this disease in history. Although only about a hundred people were acutely ill with a variety of the usual textbook symptoms, investigators suggested that somewhere between 2,894 and 7,718 people were infected.

For every disease, only a small proportion of those who are infected go to physicians, get a diagnosis, and appear in the official reporting system. This under-reporting varies between diseases and from country to country. Even in the most technologically advanced countries, the ratio of reported to actual can range from one in two to one in thousands. The degree of under-reporting is estimated from expensive, intensive follow-up of outbreaks, comparing how many people were reported initially with how many are uncovered through the intensive surveillance. There is a large margin of error in these estimates, as they are usually derived from several studies in different jurisdictions—hence the range in the estimates of the size of the B.C. epidemic. As soon as the size of the outbreak became apparent, physicians started a massive screening program for pregnant women and newborns.

After ruling out every other possible source of infection, investigators studied maps of the cases and realized that most of the infected people lived in a part of Victoria that got its water from the Humpback Reservoir. When they looked closer, they found that clusters of cases were preceded by heavy rainfall and turbid water from the reservoir and that people who drank more reservoir water were more likely to get the infection. But investigators could never prove definitively where the Victoria outbreak came from; they didn't even suspect the water until three months after the last case was detected. Still, that scenario best explained the data.

The water supply, they think, was contaminated either by wild cougars or by a profligacy of feral cats. *Toxoplasma* will have sex in any type of cat anywhere in the world, so it is no surprise that investigators found it in both feral domestic cats and cougars in the water reservoir serving Victoria. In a kind of Southern Hemisphere counterpoint to the Victoria outbreak, several hundred people in the Brazilian town of Santa Isabel do Ivai came down with toxoplasmosis in 2001. In that case, the most plausible story was that a cat gave birth to three kittens near one of the town's reservoir tanks; the kittens took up residence on the roof of the reservoir, and heavy summer rains washed the kitty poop into the water supply. People who drank the water, or ate ice cream made from the water, got sick.

There is no single, correct response to epidemics like this. If you are a cat owner who believes that un-neutered cats running free are natural and therefore good, you will likely think the cougar was the culprit in Victoria and might recommend fencing in the reservoir. If you are a wildlife biologist who believes that feral cats are a destructive, invasive species, you may recommend trapping and shooting free-running domestic cats. If you are a public health specialist—and considering the case in Brazil and the behavior of cats—you might be forgiven for thinking that there is unlikely to be a permanent solution but that public investment in protecting reservoirs and catchment areas might shift the odds against the disease.

In some ways, the prevention of direct disease transmission from pets to people seems simple and painless: get pets vaccinated and dewormed, don't let cats hunt in the wild, enforce laws that require owners to take their animal poop home with them, and wash your hands after handling an animal and before eating. Keep your dog on a leash when in public places.

But what might, from a normal scientific point of view and within household and community confines, seem a simple problem with straightforward solutions becomes much more complex when the interactions between ecology, culture, and health are accounted for. I recently visited a sheep farm that had about twenty lovely gray cats slinking around, sleeping on the sheep. The cats, I was told, were there to catch mice that would eat grain intended for the sheep, and to eat placentas after the lambs were born. If the cats weren't there, the farmer would have a problem with biological waste disposal and with mice eating feed intended for sheep. It wasn't as if you could solve the problem by saying not to keep cats.

In Europe, as in Nepal and India, dogs are everywhere, inside and outside cafés and restaurants and bake shops (as are the parasites they carry). In North America, people (myself included) often keep cats because of their pseudo-semi-wild nature and their lack of dog-like cloying dependence on people. So putting a cat on a leash defeats the purpose of having a cat and may foster an unrealistic vision of our ability to tame nature, which may be translated by policymakers into ecologically catastrophic wildlife management schemes. (As I look at the above sentence, I also realize that people, myself included, are willing to go to great lengths to justify irrational behavior.)

In North America, bites are probably the biggest threat to the public from dogs and cats. Although the fear of being bitten may draw on the deep scar left by rabies in the human psyche, the risks associated with bites are not—in North America at least—related primarily to rabies.

When I was just a little younger and still had illusions of immortality, I would sometimes go jogging in the evening to prod my body into going the distance with me. On one such evening, as I jogged through the gentle fog of a Vancouver school yard, I noticed out of the corner of my eye that an elderly gentleman was walking his dog across the shadows of the baseball diamond. What I did not see, until the dog had sunk his teeth through my trousers, was that the dog was not on a leash.

In 1994, about 4.7 million people were bitten by dogs in the United States; of these, more than 300,000 ended up in hospital emergency rooms. This is a lot, but we should keep in mind that there are about 68 million pet dogs in the United States. Most bites are about as serious as the annoying nip I suffered, but a fair proportion end up in emergency rooms. A few—about 17 every year in the U.S.—end in death. Most of the more serious bites are sustained by children under fourteen. Kids haven't learned the rules of interspecies interaction very well and may become the objects of displaced aggression when they get into the middle of a dogfight or among male dogs going after a bitch in heat, or they may be perceived by the dog as a threat to other members of the dog's pack (that is, the adopted human family).

Most incidents of dogs biting people are, from the dog's point of view, understandable. The dog is simply responding to behavioral imperatives dictated by belonging to a human pack: what's bigger than you is the boss, what's littler is to be hauled into line; protect your pack; protect your home territory. If your natural behavior is frustrated, sublimate. For most dogs, these are the rules—*unless they are trained to act otherwise.* Thus, when I was investigating a rabies epidemic in Java, I found that young boys tended to be the ones most often bitten. These would be the members of the pack in a most ambiguous position, not quite dominant and perhaps a rival. Studies in some countries have found that kids are bitten in late afternoon when they are on their way home from school and may be rowdy, and the dogs are both hungry and short-tempered after an interrupted afternoon nap.

Although I will not suggest a specific school of thought on training and restraint of dogs for fear of becoming embroiled in a battle of pedagogic ideologies, it seems to me, as a North American, that having a dog respond to a leash or training it to respond invariably to commands is essential for dogs and humans to enjoy a healthy life together. It's a bit like training children in the social graces.

Some of my friends in Kathmandu would no doubt disagree. Some of their dogs act as community police, frightening thieves away at night. What good is a community police dog on a leash? The more important underlying principle is that there are clear rules for dog-human interaction that both parties need to know. Dogs do not respond well to anarchy or to having the normal rules interfered with. Children may become injured, for instance, when they get in the way of dogs that are keyed up to fight or mate, and mountain hikers in Nepal have been attacked when they approach villages unexpectedly or after dark.

Cats attack people much more rarely and usually with less serious consequences. But a good cat scratch, claws fresh from the litter box, can result in swollen lymph glands and fever ("cat scratch fever"), and a bite can inject you with an armful of cat-mouth bacteria. Although a house cat is less inclined to pay attention to disciplinary training than a dog, how a cat is brought up and socialized has very important consequences for how it relates to other living beings.

Apart from rabies, only a few zoonoses are transmitted from companion animals to people through bites, and they are sufficiently rare to be left to medical journals and textbooks. Infections transmitted by fleas, ticks, or other biting arthropods, or from environmental contamination, however, are more common. The diseases transmitted through environmental contamination include a variety of parasites.

Roundworms (*Toxocara canis* and *Toxocara cati*) are common in puppies and kittens. The dog parasites are thought to be the most common and the most important as a source of human disease. The roundworms do their sexual-reproductive thing in the puppy intestine. The puppies can get it from their mothers; when the bitch gets pregnant, roundworm larvae in her tissues mobilize and head across the placenta and out through her milk. When she cleans her pups after birth, she may reinfect herself.

For the parasite, it's a great system, evolved over many thousands of years. A female roundworm can put out more than

100,000 eggs per day. A tangled bundle of those roundworms, which cause puppies intestinal discomfort, can put out 300,000 eggs per ounce of feces. The eggs develop best at between 50 and 86 degrees Fahrenheit and become infective after a couple of weeks, but they can survive for up to a year under a protective layer of snow or feces and still be viable.

In this way, an individual infection, if mishandled (by not enforcing pooper-scooper laws or not treating dogs with anti-parasitic drugs), can easily become a community problem. Children, exploring their surroundings through taste, may find themselves explored by nature's little visitors. If eaten, larvae of dog and cat roundworms will wander around in the human body, obviously lost in this cavernous wilderness of unfamiliar flesh, sometimes coming out the eye, where they are called ocular larva migrans, or ending up in other organs, where they are called visceral larva migrans. Many (anywhere from 8 to 63 percent) of playgrounds in North America, Europe, and Japan, as well as many backyards, have been shown to be seeded with eggs. The contamination rates in yards are not related to whether or not one owns a dog. Dogs wander and poop where they like.

In North America, where there is some modest control over dogs, scientists tend to think of this as a disease of children in unclean environments. This is not so everywhere in the world. A 1987 study in the Midi-Pyrenees region of France uncovered several dozen adults with weakness, rash, breathing trouble, and various allergic-like reactions. The researchers suggested that the disease was a "new disease syndrome" associated with visceral larva migrans and that the people had probably picked up the disease from their hunting dogs. The larvae from a variety of roundworms, however, can cause similar problems in people. In some parts of the world, these may be pig roundworms.

Domestic dogs and cats are not the only urban animals that carry zoonotic parasites. Urban centers have provided wonderful housing and free food for raccoons in North America, and rabies,

though at the top of the list of worries about these waddling suburbanites, is not the only disease on the list. Besides some afflictions that are uniquely their own, raccoons also harbor a species
of roundworms called *Baylisascaris procyonis*. Wildlife disease
experts suspect that 70 to 90 percent of raccoons might carry
these roundworms.

Children interact with their environments by tasting them,
or by crawling through them and then putting their fingers into
their mouths. Hence they are at greater risk for acquiring any diseases transmitted through environmental contamination. When
children eat the infective eggs with which the raccoons have fertilized the environment, the lost roundworm larvae sometimes
migrate to the brain. A 2005 newspaper report from Toronto
described a seven-and-a-half-year-old who suffered severe brain
damage even as perplexed physicians kept him in quarantine and
ran all kinds of tests, including an uninformative CAT scan. Not
until blood and fluid samples were tested at a veterinary laboratory at Purdue University could they make a final diagnosis. The
boy survived but is on long-term therapy and rehabilitation. In
North America, there have been more than a dozen known
deaths from this disease, but because doctors tend not to look for
it, and because there aren't any readily available, reliable tests
for it, no one knows how many people are out there with raccoon
roundworm larvae wandering around in their bodies.

Several of the bugs that give dogs or cats the trots can make
people quite sick as well. A 1984 study of *Campylobacter* infection (which causes bloody diarrhea) in college students in Geor-
gia found that eating chicken and owning cats were the main risk
factors. It should go without saying (but it doesn't, believe me)
that an animal with diarrhea should not play with little children
or visit a nursing home.

The small risk of disease and injury that a pet may pose
should not scare us away from our fellow creatures, any more
than influenza or AIDS should drive us away from the company

of other humans. For most of us, the *health* benefits of cavorting with dogs and cats far outweigh any *disease* risks. Reckless love of animals, like reckless love of the earth or of other people, carries with it natural consequences. What these diseases are telling us is that we need to "care" for each other, in the best sense of that word. To do that well, we need to gain a better understanding of the complex ecological and social roles that companion animals play, carefully managing the risks they pose even as we value their benefits.

I recall my nine-year-old son, Matthew, and me crying over the death of a young guinea pig and then, together, carrying out a post-mortem to see why it had died. Having ascertained that the cause was pneumonia, we could bury the creature in a little grave and put this knowledge to some use in how we cared for the next one. The tensions between life and death, body and spirit, eating and sacrifice, individual and group, predator and prey underlie an ecologically based ethic.

Companion animals present us with a microcosm of the inherent contradictions between health and disease; they carry parasites and microbes that could make us sick even as they lower our blood pressure and make us feel happy.

If these animals, many of whom have accompanied humanity on our long evolutionary journey from Africa, can help us to realize that we are but one of the multiple voices of nature, and that every social act is also an ecological act with possible disease-causing consequences, then they will have done us a great service. We may, after all, be remembered as part of a bright and motley choir of many species, from snow leopards, quaggas, aurochs, white-footed field mice, cicadas, cows, mosquitoes, poodles and pot-bellied pigs to Carolina parakeets singing in this small, pale sphere of light, our song an aurora borealis shimmering across the vast darkness of the universe.

(14)

POKER PLAYERS' PNEUMONIA

*T*HREE OR four times a week, eight men and four women gathered for a few hours in the small room, playing poker, drinking beer, talking. From a social-health viewpoint, this group could be seen as exemplary: not only did it include members of both genders, but also some were of Caucasian and some of African heritage. They were clearly building a social support group (what the World Bank likes to call "social capital"), and there is good evidence that communities with a lot of social capital also tend to have better health.

That winter of 1987 in Halifax, Nova Scotia, the poker players didn't pay much attention to the cat until Valentine's Day, when she gave birth to three mewling kittens. That was pretty cool. One of the kittens died, but these things happen. That's why cats have more than one in a litter and more than one litter in a lifetime. In so-called r/K selection theory, "r" strategists produce a lot of offspring and hope that some of them survive, and "K" strategists produce one or two and protect them with their lives; I would put cats slightly toward the "r" side (although not so far in that direction as, say, spiders).

On March 5, the cat's owner got sick. Over the next couple of weeks the rest of the poker group came down with cough, chest pain, sore throat, nausea, vomiting, diarrhea, and, not surprisingly, fatigue. Eleven of them got better either spontaneously (perhaps because of the beneficial effects on the immune system of good social capital) or after medical treatment with antibiotics (which the World Bank might call human capital, and which we use when the social capital fails). One person, who had a heart problem to begin with, died. Joanne Langley, Thomas Marrie, and the other epidemiologists at Dalhousie University who investigated the outbreak and reported it in the *New England Journal of Medicine* dubbed it poker players' pneumonia.

The disease that attacked the poker players is more widely known in the medical community as Q fever, a less interesting and less informative moniker. This is the kind of name given to a disease or agent when investigators don't have a clue what they are dealing with; thus, aflatoxin poisoning in England was first called turkey-X disease, and the strain of hantavirus that laid low the Navajo in the Four Corners region of the American Southwest was called *sin nombre* (no-name). The name Q fever came from Australian physician Edward H. Derrick, who in 1935 investigated an outbreak of fever in abattoir workers in Brisbane, Queensland.

According to his colleague Macfarlane Burnet, who with David White later wrote the classic book *The Natural History of Infectious Disease,* Derrick rejected the name "abattoirs fever" because it might reflect poorly on the meat industry. He couldn't use "X-disease" because it was already in use. Burnet suggested "Queensland rickettsial fever," but this was rejected because it was considered derogatory to Queensland. Derrick finally settled on "Q" for "query" fever.

As part of his investigations, Derrick injected blood and urine from sick workers into guinea pigs, who, as stalwart pawns in the army against disease, also got sick. Unable to isolate any agent, Derrick took a saline emulsion of sick–guinea pig liver and sent it to Burnet in Melbourne. Burnet, later to win the 1960 Nobel

Prize in Physiology or Medicine for his work in immunology, isolated the tiny organisms. They looked, he thought, a lot like rickettsia, which are somewhere between bacteria and viruses in size and prefer the comfort of living inside cells to the rough-and-tumble life in the free world. If they were capable of thinking and writing, one might suggest they first penned the words later paraphrased by the poet Leonard Cohen, that the cell-free life might look like freedom, but it feels like death. If, as Lynn Margulis has suggested, we are communities of bacteria, Cohen's lyrics take on a new layer of meaning.

At about the time Burnet was ferreting out the tiny organisms in Australia, Herald Cox and Gordon Davis at the Rocky Mountain Laboratory in Montana were studying ticks and the organisms they carried to try to understand two other zoonoses, Rocky Mountain spotted fever and tularemia, the latter a plague-like disease also called rabbit fever and deerfly fever, caused by a bacterium, *Francisella tularensis*, and transmitted to people through ticks, deerflies, or direct contact. A rare disease (about a hundred cases in the U.S. per year), tularemia is now considered a potential bio-terrorist agent, which to me indicates an unprecedented level of paranoia. Cox claimed to have cultivated rickettsiae from the ticks, but Dr. Rolla Dyer, director of the National Institutes of Health, was skeptical. Dyer visited Cox to challenge him and came down with fever, chills, sweats, and pain behind the eyeball (retro-orbital pain). In one of those rare instances where poetic justice does occur, blood from Dyer also made the guinea pigs sick. After the usual chaotic name calling that characterizes much microbial classification, investigators seem to have settled on the names *Coxiella burnetii* for the organism and coxiellosis for the disease (although "Q fever" is still widely used). Q fever is now reported from Uruguay to Portugal, from Russia to Australia, from Canada to China, from Switzerland to anywhere there are sheep and dust.

What was peculiar about the work of Thomas Marrie and his

friends in Nova Scotia was that the disease was associated with cats. I have a paper in my files (somewhere) that reports quite definitively that cats do not get Q fever. I also have notes from veterinary school that say quite definitely that prions do not cross the species barrier, demonstrating not that such pronouncements prove science to be a bad thing but that science does progress and that scientists should be circumspect in their pronouncements. In this way, however, scientists are at a disadvantage against the pope, archbishops, grand ayatollahs, rabbinical teachers, Pat Robertson, Billy Graham, and the presidents of the United States and Iran, who appear to have all the final answers.

Marrie went on to investigate the disease in the Maritimes and to review what is known globally about this zoonotic condition. He discovered that about 20 percent of community-acquired pneumonia in rural Nova Scotia was related to cat exposure, but he also investigated an outbreak related to skinning (dead, of course) wild rabbits. According to his team, almost half the snowshoe hares in the region had antibodies to *Coxiella burnetii*. One might suggest "wild-rabbit-skinning disease" as a good name, so as not to unfairly denigrate poker players or cats, but "Q fever," being shorter and more neutral, may be less open to the political vagaries of public language.

Sheep and goats are considered the most common reservoirs for *C. burnetii,* and in a study our group did in Ontario in the late 1980s, we found that pretty well all flocks had some evidence of infection. Outbreaks and "abortion storms" associated with coxiella infection continue to occur in sheep and goat flocks around the world, but most animals carry the microbe without showing signs of illness.

This fact has been known for decades, and it was with some dismay and bemusement that I read reports that sheep were being taken into the Hospital for Sick Children in Toronto in the early 1980s, to be used for research. The sheep were dropped off in the basement of the nurses' residence, then carted through a tunnel into the hospital itself and taken up to the ninth floor in an elevator also used by patients, visitors, and staff. As many as twenty sheep and a few goats were up there at any given time. If the research animals needed surgery, they were taken down to the eighth floor and sometimes walked down the hall. Nobody had reported getting sick, but an investigation found at least a dozen people who had had some variation of fever, diarrhea, coughing, muscle pain, and in one case hepatitis, that could be attributed to infection with *Coxiella.* The researchers almost seemed surprised.

Not long afterward, I phoned around to medical schools in southern Ontario to find out what kinds of courses were being offered on the epidemiology of zoonoses. Several thought such a course might be a good idea and had never heard of one that had been offered at Guelph for twenty years; diseases from animals were way off the medical radar.

Not long after the investigation at Sick Kids, and at about the time an outbreak in people who had contact with sick goats at the Royal Agricultural Winter Fair in Toronto was unfolding, one of the few veterinarians in the Ontario Ministry of Health was accosted by a new, perplexed minister of health with the question: what's a veterinarian doing in the Ministry of Health? What indeed.

The late 1980s were a time of generally heightened concern (sometimes verging on panic) about Q fever and sheep. The incidents at Toronto Sick Kids and community outbreaks stimulated a review of how sheep are screened before entering research centers in Canada, including the Ontario Veterinary College, where I work. Veterinary students learn a lot of important things from sheep, although not how to panic and run at unexpected noises, which is a good thing for future clients. For four years, in parallel with the procedural changes for disease-screening experimental sheep, I ran a "blood-for-doughnuts" program. In return for doughnuts and coffee, students in one veterinary class donated blood every semester and filled in little questionnaires about exposure to animals. I followed the class from their first year all the way through to graduation, but only one or two of them showed any evidence of exposure, and that wasn't at the vet college. One could almost hear an administrative sigh of relief.

But sheep and goats aren't the only reservoirs, as Thomas Marrie demonstrated. One of my late colleagues in Ontario, Gerhard Lang, who himself suffered from a chronic form of Q fever, found widespread evidence of exposure to the agent in cattle as well. There is evidence that infected cattle can shed it in their milk for more than two years, but, although the cattle in Ontario had antibodies, indicating that they had been exposed, there was no evidence that they were actively infected.

Scientists don't have a very good idea which animals might be carrying and shedding the organism; it is very infectious at small doses (one organism is apparently enough to make a person sick), and laboratory technicians are not keen to work with it. Researchers are therefore left with secondary evidence, such as antibodies in serum, which indicate that the animals were once exposed to the organisms but don't say much about current infection or shedding.

In the absence of abortions and stillbirths in animals, there is not much to go on, either in animals or people. Clinical signs (things that can be seen and measured, such as temperature) and symptoms (things that are felt, such as pain and headaches) aren't unique to Q fever. The disease also varies from place to place, probably depending on particular strains of the organism. In the Maritimes of Canada, pneumonia seems to be the main disease; in other places, it is hepatitis, diarrhea, or general "flu-like" syndromes, which is why it is not surprising that the hospital-infection-control people in Toronto had not detected an outbreak until after it had occurred. Chronically, the coxiella can stick to heart valves and cause a debilitating endocarditis.

I have left one question hanging in the air: how do people get the disease from animals? In the summer of 1981, twenty-nine people in Gwent, south Wales, came down with fever, severe headaches, and malaise. "Malaise" is a technical term for feeling bummed out, under the weather. (I sometimes ponder, as a specialist in zoonoses, what wonderful afflictions I might be suffering. Alas, I suspect my malaise has more to do with new headlines from the Middle East than bacteria, viruses, or rickettsia.) Two of those afflicted in Gwent county developed something considerably more serious than my middle-class, hypochondriac whinging: hepatitis and endocarditis. The person with the infected valves died, and the cause of death was demonstrated by infecting and then sacrificing a guinea pig; those who say animal sacrifice is obsolete little know the costs of our well-being and scientific knowledge. Investigators followed every possible lead as to how people got infected. In the end, they decided that farm trucks had driven through the neighborhood, stirring up clouds of contaminated straw and manure.

At least the good people in the villages of Val de Bagnes in Valais Canton, Switzerland, enjoyed the pleasures of watching sheep, and not just ramshackle trucks, flock down their valley from mountain pastures to market. The autumn of 1983 was an especially dry one, and over four hundred villagers came down with Q fever. About half the people had shivering, severe headaches, severe exhaustion, and loss of appetite. Some of them had more severe chest pains, coughs, dizziness, and abdominal pains.

According to the investigators, "More than half of the patients suffering from Q fever were not seen by a doctor, being either only slightly ill or not ill at all." This is an interesting use of the word "suffering," which I shall have to keep in mind when tallying up a lifetime of such afflictions. On the plus side, the researchers made the remarkable suggestion that physicians and veterinarians talk to each other and perhaps even work together. After decades of resistance, diseases such as Q fever, avian influenza, and West Nile virus have encouraged some movement in that direction.

What almost all the outbreaks have in common is that fluids and materials from animals that have recently given birth spill into the environment, dry up, and get blown around by the wind. They are tough and can survive a long time under difficult environmental conditions. Near Aix-en-Provence, France, investigators attributed higher rates of the disease to a local wind, the mistral, which came down from the northwest and passed over a sheep-rearing area before entering the small town of Martigues; the pristine air of southern France was harboring more than romance for starry-eyed tourists. Some cases have been traced to drinking infected milk, but I suspect that the milk splashed and people breathed in the fresh, warm, down-home scent of infection. One version of the infection cycle shows *Coxiella burnetii* being transmitted from wild animals to people and domestic animals by ticks, which, given all the other bad stuff ticks carry, should not be surprising.

In 1978, four employees of an "exotic bird and reptile importing company" in New York State were set back with the usual fever, chills, and severe headaches. They had been unpacking and deticking a shipment of five hundred ball pythons (*Python reguis*); the ticks were carrying *Coxiella burnetii*. Carriage by ticks is not thought to be common, but then who would have thought pythons were pets? The people who shipped the snakes from some tropical country must have shaken their heads in wonder; maybe they thought Americans eat them? The traffic in such so-called exotic pets is one of the most efficient ways for strange diseases to travel the globe.

In Poland, epidemiological patterns and experiments in mice suggested the possibility of sexual transmission, which could lead to all manner of inappropriate jokes. But I suppose most infections can be spread that way, depending on how one defines "sex."

BANG'S DISEASE

AND THE WHITE PLAGUE

*T*HIS SECTION on zoonoses that people acquire from our closest companions would not be complete without considering two of the oldest and deadliest diseases associated with domestic livestock: Bang's disease (brucellosis) and the white plague (tuberculosis).

Diseases caused by mycobacteria, a family that includes leprosy as well as various forms of tuberculosis, are among the most ancient of zoonoses. Spinal damage typical of some forms of tuberculosis has been found in Egyptian mummies from as far back as four thousand to five thousand years ago.

When leprosy all but disappeared from Europe after the Black Death swept through in the mid-fourteenth century, its sister, tuberculosis, appeared to rise up in a wave and displace it, peaking among the ill-housed and ill-fed industrial workers in the nineteenth century, dropping well before Robert Koch discovered the tubercle bacillus, and continuing to drop as nutrition and housing improved in the early twentieth century, partly in response to the bacteriological discoveries of people like Koch and Louis Pasteur.

Drugs and vaccines provided the tools to finally get rid of it, but TB dug in and held on in areas of poverty and overcrowding, saved in part by misguided politicians and physicians, who now saw diseases as *only* medical problems and therefore saw no need to work for improving social conditions as a fundamental condition for good health. More recently, concurrent with the collapse of the Soviet Union and the general skepticism among international financial institutions and development donors toward government-sponsored health-and-welfare programs, and along with the spread of AIDS in fragmented economies and marginalized populations, the old white plague is making a comeback.

Now, every year, some eight million people—many in sub-Saharan Africa, many with concurrent HIV infection—come down with tuberculosis; a couple of million people a year die.

Tuberculosis has a complex social and ecological history. The disease conjures for some the romantic "consumption" of nineteenth-century wraiths and doe-eyed poets. Others think of sanitariums where tubercular people retreated for fresh air in the first part of the twentieth century—now long gone or used as retreats for aspiring writers. Others recall the image of a foolhardy and compassionate Dr. Norman Bethune, kissing a woman with TB so that she could feel some human warmth before she died.

Except for veterinarians, few people think of tuberculosis as a zoonosis. In 1901, Koch stated absolutely that tuberculosis could never be transmitted from cattle to people, and that public health measures to prevent such transmission were ill-advised. He held to this position in the face of a great deal of contrary evidence. Much to the dismay of some veterinary scientists, such as Daniel Elmer Salmon (after whom *Salmonella* was named), who was the director of the U.S. Bureau of Animal Industry, Koch's arguments were used to support the sale of meat and milk from animals with TB.

In the next few decades, investigators from the Ministry of Agriculture in the United Kingdom demonstrated that 40 percent of dairy cattle in that country were tuberculous, and that

2,500 people per year, most of them children under five, were
dying from bovine tuberculosis.

The pulmonary form of the disease with which many of us
are familiar, in which the lungs are invaded and victims cough
and spit blood, is transmitted by people spraying bacteria at
each other. However, tuberculosis of the bones and intestinal
tracts, which is more common in younger people and in developing countries, probably comes from ingestion of organisms
through food and could well be from cattle. Scientists don't usually know which TB is coming from people and which from other
animals; even when TB is diagnosed, the countries where it is
most common don't have the facilities to differentiate among the
various strains.

The findings from the U.K. in the early twentieth century
stimulated disease eradication programs in cattle. Along with
test-and-slaughter programs, in which infected animals (or
infected herds) were slaughtered, the advent of pasteurization all
but eliminated this route of infection in industrialized countries.
However, the disease is still widespread in cattle (and other species) in many poor southern countries.

Mycobacteria are still pretty much everywhere, albeit in scattered pockets of poverty or wilderness. In North America, bison
and elk are known to be infected. Besides *Mycobacterium bovis*
and *M. tuberculosis, M. avium* occurs in a wide range of birds, as
well as in pigs, cattle, deer—and in people with AIDS. One strain,
M. marinum, is found in fish. In the United Kingdom and Ire-
land, badgers are infected with *M. Bovis,* and in New Zealand,
brushtail possums (*Trichosurus vulpecula*), ferrets, wild deer,
and wild pigs. There is also evidence that dogs, cats, and parrots
can get TB from people or cattle.

Given the widespread wildlife reservoirs, the difficulty in
treating TB (six months of daily, expensive treatments with some
potentially toxic drugs), the pandemic of AIDS (about 10 percent

of TB globally is in people with AIDS), and the lack of political will to tackle difficult problems of economic disparity, TB is likely to be with us just about as long as we ourselves manage to stay around. The vaccine, BCG—bacillus Calmette-Guérin, named for the French scientists who developed it—is of uncertain efficacy; originally derived from cattle TB by a veterinarian and a physician, ironically it is even less effective in cattle than in people.

Brucellosis is probably not as old as TB, but a disease that causes abortion in animals and fevers in people is difficult to distinguish from the background noise of the aches and pains of our normal mortal coil. There is archaeological evidence of brucellosis cases going back to the fourth millennium BC in Italy, Egypt, and the Near East, and to 400–230 BC in pre-Roman Britain. Since goats—one of the animal reservoirs for this disease—have been domesticated for about nine thousand years, this news should not be surprising. Also, since the disease was known locally in many areas before anyone knew exactly what caused it, we should not be surprised that it goes by many names: Cyprus fever, undulating fever, Malta fever, Mediterranean fever, relapsing fever, rock fever, and Bang's disease.

The bacterium that causes brucellosis was isolated in 1887 by David Bruce in Malta. Bruce, also of *Trypanosoma brucei* fame, was investigating Mediterranean fever, first described by Hippocrates in 450 BC and in the nineteenth century a problem for the Royal Navy. The disease was a chronic, debilitating condition affecting Royal Navy seamen (and other local people, but, as ever, it was the warriors who "mattered"). Themistocles Zammit, a Maltese physician-archaeologist and a member of the British government commission run by Bruce, discovered the natural host for the disease. In the fashion of all good scientists, Zammit made his discovery serendipitously: He was planning to use goats as experimental animals, since they didn't seem to get sick from the organism. Raw goats' milk had, until then (and in many places, until now), sometimes been used to help patients in the hospital get well. Zammit demonstrated the organism in the milk of apparently healthy goats. Bruce called the bug *Micrococcus melitensis*. This organism, later renamed *Brucella melitensis,* is found almost entirely in goats and in people who handle aborted goat fetuses or drink raw milk or eat fresh cheese made from milk from infected goats. Aging cheese kills a lot of bacteria, as the cheese gets more acidic over time.

In 1897, Danish veterinarian Bernhard Bang found a similar organism, which eventually was christened with the somewhat less mellifluous name *Brucella abortus.* At least two others are now recognized: *B. suis,* found in pigs, hares, reindeer, musk oxen, and caribou, and *B. canis,* found in, well, canines.

The disease in people can start weeks to months after they have ingested the organisms and can include any or all or none of fever, sweats, depression, headache, backache, vomiting, diarrhea or constipation, certain kinds of arthritis—especially sacroileitis—and heart, lung, and urinary tract problems. In animals, the organism causes abortion in females and inflammation of the joints and genital organs in males. It can settle into udders and lymph nodes and be excreted with the animal showing few signs of illness.

The tactics used to get rid of brucellosis have been very similar to those for TB. In this case, the eradication programs had the head start of a good live vaccine—good enough not only to protect cows, but also to infect a lot of veterinarians who accidentally injected themselves while trying to jab the unhappy cattle. Once the level of disease had been decreased through vaccination, livestock farmers could push through with a test-and-slaughter policy.

As for TB, pasteurization all but eliminated brucellosis in people except for abattoir workers, farmers, veterinarians, and all those hundreds of millions of people around the world who like raw goats' milk and fresh goat cheese, or who can't afford or who don't have access to pasteurization or firewood for cooking the milk. Also, as for TB, wildlife reservoirs persist.

In Canada and the United States, from at least the late 1980s on, various scientists, advocacy groups, and politicians wrestled with what to do about infections with *B. abortus* in wild wood bison in Wood Buffalo National Park in northern Alberta and bison and elk in Yellowstone National Park. "Solutions" have ranged from killing all the bison and putting in "clean" ones, to carrying out some kind of test-and-slaughter program, to building fences around areas the size of Switzerland, to doing nothing. The kill-all-and-repopulate strategy (which many cattle ranchers supported) raises a lot of hackles, given how poorly we understand even the simplest ecosystems. First Nations groups in Canada are skeptical of government intentions and suspect the disease problem is being exaggerated. Up to 2006, the do-nothing side seemed to be winning. It is not clear that brucellosis has any impact on the bison populations; although a female may abort in her first year, she is okay (and immune) in years after that.

In the U.S., hunters and outfitters have supported the setting up of feeding grounds for elk, but those also provide increased opportunity for diseases to spread. Bison and cattle don't mix much, and some have suggested that vaccinating the bison could get rid of the disease, as long as the elk populations were allowed to fall back to "natural" numbers (no feeding grounds).

When the issue first hit the headlines, I remember some people arguing that we absolutely had to do something, and we had to do it soon, or else... I don't remember where the "or else" led, but probably to reinfected cattle herds and loss of international trade, plus dire public health consequences. But no politician could stomach a public massacre of bison, so the "problem" was left. Both TB and brucellosis shuffle around in these populations, spread, and probably infect some people—hunters, mostly.

How important is brucellosis? It depends on what criteria you are using. Who gets sick is as important as how many. As historian William McNeill points out in *Plagues and Peoples,* epidemics among armies have changed the course of political and military history. So the British had good cause to be concerned.

Sometimes one case has amazing implications. I recently visited the Sagrada Familia ("Holy Family") basilica in Barcelona, Spain, the organic, wildly celebratory work by the Catalan modernist architect Antoni Gaudí. According to some of his associates, Gaudi lived on a spartan diet of olive oil, nuts, lettuce, chard, bread with honey, and a few splashes of goats' milk. In 1911, the splashes of milk caught up with him in the form of a severe bout of brucellosis. This chronically debilitating disease was one of the influences that led him to set aside all other projects and focus exclusively on what was to become his (unfinished) masterpiece, the Sagrada Familia. Without the disease, would the world be culturally poorer?

In the U.S., there are maybe a hundred human cases a year. In Canada, there are far fewer. Brucellosis is described as being "endemic" in parts of Africa, Latin America, the Mediterranean, and Asia, but "endemic" in this case can refer to anything from less than 0.01 sick people per 100,000 to over 200 per 100,000.

No doubt the effects outside North America are far greater than within. It seems to me that the angry passion attached to the debate in North America and the drastic "solutions" proposed are in inverse proportion to the seriousness of the disease. There are programmatic costs—maintaining a surveillance system and trained laboratory personnel—to maintaining a situation where there is always some risk, where the disease is not eradicated, where the bacteria live on in pockets of wildlife, but those are the costs of living in a complex, beautiful, amazing, heartbreaking planet. That's gotta be worth a few bucks.

(16)

DOG PARASITES IN THE
LAND OF THE GODS

*L*IKE MANY westerners, I found enlightenment in Kathmandu. My gurus were a tapeworm and a Nepalese veterinarian.

I arrived in Nepal, for the third time in my life, on the thirteenth day of the month of Mangshir, 2049. I thought, in my Western naivete, that it was November 28, 1992. But our calendars, whether Julian (Western) or Bikram Sambat (Nepalese), were largely irrelevant.

Crossing the footbridge over the Bishnumati River in the chill, dark predawn, I could see a series of fires on the far bank, men and dark shapes of water buffalo appearing and disappearing as the light flickered, a scene from summer camp or Dante's hell.

As our little coterie of scientists drew closer, we could see several men grappling with one of the beasts, hammering a long, blood-covered spike into the base of the buffalo's skull. The buffalo sank into a bed of straw on the ground as one of the men moved in to slit the throat and get a good blood flow. The man stood up to stretch his back, wiping his bloody hands on his jeans. He was in a winter jacket with a turned-back wool collar and big rubber boots. The men piled straw over the body and fanned it into flames to burn off the coarse black hair, then stood back to watch. When the fires died down, they rolled the stiffening body on to its back, and one of them leaned down to slit open the belly. One man, who was barefoot, his loose slacks rolled up to the knees, stepped forward to pull the great, bulging white, blood-flecked rumen out of the body cavity. Another, in a red sleeveless shirt, sweatpants, and a woolen toque, cut open the chest cavity and pulled out the heart and lungs. The team of young men waded around in the spilled guts, stomach contents, and shit, steam rising into the chilled air around them as they quietly went about the work of preparing meals for tourists and other wealthy consumers.

I rubbed my hands together to keep the blood flowing and zipped my windbreaker closed over my heavy sweater. As morning light exhaled and condensed down from the snowy peaks and across the valley, dogs and pigs nosed in and out of the fading darkness at the periphery of this tableau, repeated every few dozen yards along the riverbank.

Scanning the scene before me, I wondered what the big black lumps were on the branches of the huge trees stretching up from the muck. Fruiting bodies of some sort, I thought. One of them stretched his wings and glided away. They were vultures, I realized with a shudder, hundreds of them, and a giant murder of crows, thousands of them. Our guide through this world of blood and shadows was Dr. D.D. Joshi, soon to be friend and colleague, a Nepalese veterinarian with a passionate dedication to improving the lives of his compatriots. He loosened the scarf around his neck, tucked back the sleeve of his white shirt, and pointed to the riverbank beside us, where piles of buffalo feet, manure, blood, and offal spilled down in an inchoate mess to the small black trickle, which was all that was left of the river. Ducks, pigs, and dogs foraged for maggots and bits of discarded bone and fat, and, down by the thin stream of water through the muck, men and women defecated and washed.

"There used to be broad, stone stairs down to the river here," Joshi said. "Somewhere underneath all that . . . " He waved his hand. "People would go down for their morning ablutions."

We stepped up the steeply sloped alleys away from the main slaughtering area, past several groups of buffalo awaiting the knife. Kids clambered over them; this was the youngsters' playground. We walked the alleys, noting a flow of dogs toward the slaughtering areas at the riverside and the curious pattern of how some groups of dogs would reach a cross-street and then stop, as if held back by some invisible force. We collected dog shit in little film containers and marked the slaughtering places on our tourist maps of Kathmandu. A little way up a narrow, potholed alley, the medieval, delicately carved wooden balconies leaning over us, we looked into a dank doorway. Inside, on a bed of filthy straw, several men were cutting up a carcass.

"Female buffaloes get killed inside," said Dr. Joshi. "It's illegal to kill females of breeding age. The government wants to ensure that there are enough work animals in the countryside." He didn't have to add that farmers will do what they have to do, cull the sick or lame, sell to make ends meet. But knowing me—knowing westerners—he did add: "Of course, we don't kill cows, only buffaloes, because of their different religious significance."

As we continued upward toward a small intersection, we passed a wall covered with half-dried pancakes of cow dung. Once dried, these burn with almost no smell, an important source of cooking fuel in a country with no oil reserves and an increasingly deforested countryside. The city was beginning to wake up. Inside houses everywhere, I could hear hacking and coughing and lung clearing. A great gob of phlegm was lobbed out a shop door past me and into the street. I recalled that lower respiratory disease and tuberculosis were both on the top ten killer list globally and were common in Nepal. A few seconds later, a woman in a well-worn sari stepped out, looked up and down the street, smiled happily at us, and disappeared back into the darkness of her shop.

We stopped for sweet, milky Nepalese tea at the corner, cupping the glasses in our hands to warm ourselves. Wondering if the tea were hot enough to kill the bacteria in the water used to rinse the glasses between customers, I spilled a little over the lip on the side from which I planned to drink. Soon the sky had turned from gray-pink to pale blue, a mist hanging in the early morning December air, veiling the white vistas of heaven. A rickshaw was being pushed uphill past us, and we stepped out to have a look at the pile of meat spilling over its sides.

Peter Schantz, a veterinary parasitologist from the Centers for Disease Control and Prevention, pointed out a fist-sized, whitish, semi-opaque cyst in the lungs in the rickshaw. He rolled it bare-handed between his fingers. This was the parasite we—Canadian veterinarian Dominique Baronet (my graduate student), Schantz, Don de Savigny, from the International Development Research Centre in Ottawa (our funder, and a parasitologist himself), Dr. Joshi, and I—were here to understand and to do something about. There were a lot of problems associated with the dogs of Kathmandu, including rabies. But Joshi had not brought us half-way around the world to do something about rabies, as important as that was. He already knew what could be done about rabies and was already running free clinics to vaccinate dogs as often as he could get donations to do so. No, Joshi had brought us to this medieval city that was his home to help him figure out how to deal with a tapeworm of dogs.

In dogs, *Echinococcus granulosus* is a tiny, mostly harmless tapeworm. If you follow the dogs around the narrow streets of Kathmandu and carefully, painstakingly finger your way through piles of fresh feces (much to the delightful scorn of neighborhood children), or better yet (from an investigative point of view), thread your way through the yards of intestines in a freshly dead dog, you can sometimes find tiny, glistening bits of raw pasta. These are the adult tapeworms. Trying to find a living specimen is a lot like trying to find a grain of wet rice in a pile of dog feces.

Dogs pick up the infection by eating the fertile cysts of the kind we had seen in the buffalo lung; these large, fleshy balls of fluid and tapeworm heads are found in herbivorous animals of many kinds, the most important of which worldwide have been sheep. In the Arctic regions of the world, caribou, reindeer, and voles more commonly serve as intermediate hosts. The term "host" has a genteel, Emily Post resonance, as when the pathologists ask me to *appreciate* a fine lesion. But "host" refers to the larger animals on which the smaller animals (the parasites) feed.

The tapeworm is a good guest in the dog, in whom it does not appear to cause any disease or discomfort. The cysts are another matter.

Historically, as for many other multihost parasites, scientific investigators first discovered what they thought were several unrelated diseases in people and animals, each with a different story. In people, for instance, the slowly growing cyst came to be called hydatid disease. Such cysts have been described in both people and animals, going back to early naturalist-healers such as Hippocrates (third century BC), Aretaeus of Cappadocia (first century AD), and Galen (second century AD). While physicians tended to view such cysts as tumors growing spontaneously from various organs, as early as the seventeenth century some naturalists suggested similarities between the cysts in people and cysts in other animals and described what appeared to be tapeworm heads inside them.

Depending on where the cyst occurs, the clinical disease has different manifestations. Usually it settles in the liver, where, as it enlarges, it acts as a slowly growing tumor and causes abdominal discomfort. In severe cases, people look as if they are pregnant; in an alien-species-type way, they are: pregnant with thousands of tiny tapeworms. If the parasite makes a cyst in the lungs, such as the one we fondled in the rickshaw, it can result in a dry cough, or, if it ruptures, coughing of blood. One strain of the parasite that occurs in the circumpolar region of the globe and is common in some parts of Tibet and northwestern China (with a different species name, *multilocularis,* from that of the more common variety we saw in Nepal) cycles between caribou and wolves or between foxes and voles. *Echinococcus multilocularis* behaves more like a malignant tumor, sending little buds and daughter cysts around the body.

There are few good treatments for hydatid disease. Surgery to remove the cysts can be risky, for if the cyst ruptures, hundreds of tiny "daughters" are spread all through the body, sending the patient into shock and leading to death. Antiparasitic drugs, which have been tried in various combinations and for different periods of time, are only partly effective in reducing cyst size and require long-term treatment.

Dogs contaminate the environment with wiggling sections of tapeworm, each containing several hundred eggs. Intermediate hosts—sheep, goats, camels, water buffalo, swine—ingest the eggs, which (to simplify a more complicated story) slide down the esophagus and through the stomach and then migrate across the intestinal wall and through the bloodstream to some congenial resting place. There a cyst develops, within which daughter capsules bud off and little prototapeworms are formed.

This cyst stage of the parasite is not harmful to people. People could eat these cysts without becoming infected, though I don't know of any good recipes offhand. It's the dogs that get infected from the cysts. When the sheep or other host dies, and a dog or a coyote or a fox eats the viscera or is fed the cyst as waste from the slaughter, the baby parasites attach themselves to the intestinal wall and complete the life cycle.

In this cycle, people take the place of other livestock. This fact is a useful reminder, for those who might have forgotten, of our animal nature. Thus, we pick up the disease from dogs. In some cultures, such as among the Turkana people in Kenya, who live in an area where water is scarce, dogs may be used to clean off young children. Being licked by a dog might be better than no bath at all, but it can also transmit disease. In Lebanon, shoemakers once used a mixture of dog feces and water to prepare hides and thus were at special risk. Among certain groups of people in Kathmandu, Dominique Baronet discovered, dogs are valued members of the community for religious and social reasons. In many cultures, children snuggle up to dogs or play on floors in houses where dogs may have relieved themselves.

The unfortunate parasites that end up in human bodies find themselves stuck as strangers in a strange land, in what parasitologists call a dead-end host. People are not really a part of the natural maintenance cycle. In most cases, people don't reinfect dogs; that's the natural job of other livestock species. The reason for this is that we don't normally slaughter people; well, that's actually not true, although often we cremate them or make some attempt to hide the bodies after we have slaughtered them. More important, we aren't usually eaten by dogs. An exception may occur among the Turkana, who sometimes bury their dead in shallow graves and whose dogs are hungry.

But in Nepal, humans were a dead end. In a survey of local hospitals, Joshi found that more than 20 percent of people who had surgery for cyst removal died during or shortly after surgery. However common or uncommon the disease might be, the prognosis of those who got it was not good.

By the late nineteenth century, scientists were beginning to understand the complete life cycle of the parasite; today, dog, livestock, and human diseases are often referred to by the collective term "cystic echinococcosis." This parasite has a home on every continent except (possibly) Antarctica, although the prevalence varies from place to place, and a few countries have successfully eradicated it. It occurs at highest levels in parts of Africa, central Asia, and southern South America. Recently a team from

Switzerland calculated that the global burden of disease imposed by cystic echinococcosis was on the order of a billion disability-adjusted life years.

THAT DAY IN 1992, having seen the animals being slaughtered, the cysts, and the dogs, we continued up the streets behind the fires—narrow brick and potholed asphalt streets curved up between ancient brick walls and finely carved, cracked, ancient wooden balustrades. We paused at Durbar Square, an area of ancient temples, small shops, wandering tourists, open markets, and the "old" city of Kathmandu. Freak Street, which led away from the square and which I had visited as a vagabond in 1967, had slumped into a quiet backwater. The place to be now for travelers was Thamel, a twenty-minute walk from Durbar, its bustling streets crowded with restaurants, and hiking and souvenir shops, a magnet for hikers, dope dealers, carpet sellers, and seekers of enlightenment.

We circled back down the main road to the Bhimsentan Bridge. The vendors were laying out their wares on the sidewalk: brass pots, cotton shirts, and fruit. Tailors were tuning their sewing machines. Below, the pigs foraged in offal from slaughtered buffalo and open latrines. I looked up to cloud-shrouded mountains and then along the bridge. Nearby, a girl on the sidewalk very carefully stacked lychees and peaches in pyramids of five. With nimble grace and dignity, she crossed her legs and waited.

As we walked back to Joshi's office, I noticed a small, thin dog sitting on a blanket near a door. An old Gurkha dozed in the doorway. A heap of dogs lay nearby, their bodies rising and falling in peaceful sleep. A little farther along, three small boys in rags were piled up like sacks of rice, sleeping. By this time, the sun was up and the temperature rising fast. By midday it was in the mid-seventies, and we had peeled off our sweaters and were down to T-shirts.

We were gathered around a wooden table in a small room at the National Zoonoses and Food Hygiene Research Centre. The center was Joshi's modest two-story house with a large black-and-white sign at the gate. I could almost imagine that we were a revolutionary cell of scientists ready to bring hope, enlightenment, clean water, less garbage, and an animal inspection act to the dark chaos around us.

As we settled down with our tea in Dr. Joshi's house, we knew that to understand this parasitic disease we would need to do surveys of infection in livestock, in dogs, and in people. We would need to understand something of livestock movements, since many of the animals being slaughtered in the valley came from elsewhere and hence would have been infected elsewhere. We would need to understand something about how people and their dogs related to each other. In some ways, it was a relief to have all these details to focus on. These things were doable. Good basic science. And if we understood all these things, could we not also make them better? Didn't knowing the problem take us halfway to having solved it?

Later, filled with a sense of confidence and purpose, some of us (the westerners) went out to Mike's Breakfast, an open-garden restaurant near the luxurious Yak and Yeti Hotel. Mike had come from Minnesota in the 1960s as a Peace Corps volunteer and, like many others, had stayed. His restaurant was still the best place to get great coffee, yogurt, and fruit and listen to Mozart and eavesdrop on trekkers planning an ascent of Everest.

That evening, I stopped my bicycle in the middle of the bridge to gaze up the valley. I recalled a visit earlier that week with one of the keen young lions in the Ministry of Health. I was there to inform him that we had some human rabies vaccine available, not just for our researchers, but for use by Ministry of Health people in the area. He proclaimed that Nepal had its own perfectly good vaccine and that the human diploid vaccine recommended by the World Health Organization caused cancer. He seemed annoyed that we (outside scientists) were starting a research project when the answers were already obvious. The way to get rid of both rabies and hydatid disease, he said, was through mass gassing of street dogs.

I did not have the temerity to ask how this would be accomplished. I was, after all, a visitor, and his implication was that scientific imperialism had somehow insinuated itself into the niche left open by the political imperialists. The accusation had a ring of truth, and I was left feeling angry and disheartened. How did one demonstrate global solidarity without falling into the old patterns?

But now, on the bridge, in this warm, lucid light, I again felt hopeful. The sidewalks on the bridge were crowded with hawkers selling shirts, sweaters, shoes, fruits, vegetables, live chickens, and pots. Below me, the Bishnumati River snaked its dark, sluggish way between the herds of buffalo awaiting slaughter, the pigs, the dogs, people defecating, piles of offal and bones, chaos of life and death. The narrow, medieval streets of Bhimsentan rose up from this visceral chaos of life and death to the centers of commerce and contemplation at Durbar Square. And above the river itself, above the dark silhouettes of the near mountains, I caught a glimpse of the white, heavenly peaks. For no logical reason I could think of, it filled me with a sense of timelessness, peace, and hope. We would prove that Ministry of Health official wrong. There were better, more democratic, more humane ways of learning our way into a healthy future.

We were going to save wards 19 and 20 in Kathmandu. And if we could reclaim this small part of Shangri-La from the depths into which it had fallen, was there not hope for the whole world? Might there not be a path into a sustainable, healthy, convivial future?

IN JUNE 1995, as I flew into Kathmandu from Bangkok, my mental landscape was in turmoil. I had been reading a *Newsweek* article about the environmental catastrophe, the cesspool of garbage and muck that was the riverside in downtown Kathmandu, the area where my collaborators had lived and worked for the past three years. The comments of one of my Canadian colleagues back home rang in my ears: "Kathmandu is an ecological disaster, a write-off. We might as well let the place crash, and start over from the ashes." Was he right? I had been taught that epidemiology is an applied science, that the reason we went to all this effort was to solve real-world public health problems. Why hadn't the work of our research team made any discernible impact?

The science part of this equation involved gathering evidence. The applied part was to persuade policymakers to take up the knowledge we generated and use it.

We had certainly gathered evidence.

SINCE WE HAD begun our work in Kathmandu in 1992, Dominique and Dr. Joshi and the other researchers had doggedly pursued the demands of good, conventional, normal science. Working with our Nepalese colleagues, Dominique spent many hours documenting the behavior of dogs in Kathmandu and collecting fresh dog feces. She then put fluorescent collars on the dogs, took pictures of them, and injected them with vaccines for rabies and antiparasitic drugs. She developed a veritable mugs' gallery of the street dogs of Kathmandu. She not only probed through dog feces searching for those rice-grain-sized tapeworm segments but also, working with a new laboratory test, searched the feces for bits of tapeworm too small to be seen with even the best microscopes.

To do household surveys, we needed detailed street maps, which were easier described than found, given the warren of unnamed alleys and small courtyards that characterize old Kathmandu. It took major detective work and days of waiting in offices with the sunlight filtering down beams of dust to yellowing piles of paper for Dominique to get detailed city maps. At least here, in contrast to Indonesia, where I had worked previously, city maps were not considered military secrets. Based on her maps, and many days of walking the alleys of wards 19 and 20, Dominique was able to conduct a random survey of households in the area to see how people related to their dogs and to assess their knowledge of disease and hygiene.

The picture that emerged from our evidence was complicated. Our team was able to establish levels of infection (and reinfection) in dogs, livestock, and people. There were cysts in 5 to 8 percent of the buffalo, goats, and sheep slaughtered along the riverbank. Many of these animals came from India and Tibet, so the primary cycles of infection were probably in those countries. Only about 6 percent of the dogs in Kathmandu were infected, and reinfection rates were very low, suggesting that the disease was still primarily an import.

Infections in both dogs and people were not, we discovered, restricted to the butchering areas. Butchers did not trim out the hydatid cysts but sold them along with the meat, which was priced according to weight. Thus, it was the squeamish consumers who cut out the cysts and fed them to their dogs. Working with the veterinary clinics we had recruited throughout the city, we were able to identify dogs in "suburbia" that were thus infected. Many of the dogs were valued as pets or guard dogs.

About 60 percent of the dog owners in the areas where livestock were slaughtered were feeding raw meat, offal, bones, or cysts to their dogs. Unlike people in North America, where feeding raw meats to dogs has become a health-food fad, these people fed their dogs raw meat because they didn't have many alternatives. In whatever country one lives, feeding raw meat to dogs is a great way to spread all sorts of diseases from livestock to dogs and to the people handling the dog food.

Usually the work went on as expected. It was the surprises that gave some of the most useful information. While Dominique was working, some artifacts were stolen from a local temple. For some of the residents, a reasonable explanation of these events went like this: Canadian woman comes into our neighborhood, injecting dogs with strange drugs. The dogs, who are our community police, die. The thieves move in. Fortunately, Dominique had built up a lot of goodwill in the community, and we could continue our work despite the suspicions.

Another complication arose when we went through our test results from people. Although 35 to 40 percent of households in the slaughtering neighborhood had at least one person test positive on an initial screening test for *Echinococcus*, these tests were not confirmed by a second test done by the Centers for Disease Control and Prevention.

Peter Schantz suggested that maybe we were looking at another parasite, the so-called pork tapeworm, or cysticercus cellulosae in its larval form. The adult tapeworm, *Taenia solium*, inhabits the guts of people, and the bladder-like cyst housing the heads of the tapeworms lives in pigs. In poor countries throughout the world, the pigs get infected when they eat human feces, sometimes the only food available to them. Where clean water is not available, people may infect themselves, with tragic results: the cysts spin through the bloodstream throughout the body and can end up in the brain; the resulting inflammation may lead to epileptic-like seizures and psychotic-like personality changes. This disease is called neurocysticercosis. Cate Dewey, a veterinarian from Guelph, has recently been studying the connections between epilepsy and this parasite in poor villages in eastern Africa. The villagers, trying to supplement their meager farm incomes, and to support AIDS orphans and to send their children to school, had been given pigs to raise and sell. Without knowledge of the parasite, adequate feed for the pigs, or easily available clean water and latrines, the disease has become a serious burden.

Parasitologist Robert Desowitz describes an epidemic of burns among the Ekari people in what was once Western New Guinea, now called (by the Indonesians at least) Irian Jaya. The epidemic occurred several years after Western New Guinea was absorbed by Indonesia, and President Suharto's armies brought a gift of Balinese pigs to soften up the local population and prepare them for an influx of impoverished refugees from overcrowded Java. The pigs were infected with the cysts of *T. solium*. The Ekari, who were fond of quickly barbecued pork (a.k.a. slightly warmed dead pig), subsequently picked up the tapeworm. Lacking both refrigeration (which over time can kill the cysticerci) and ample clean water for washing their hands, they suffered an epidemic of neurocysticercosis; during the seizures, especially on cold nights, sufferers would stumble into the fires around which they slept.

It appeared that a similar situation could be unfolding in Nepal, given the widespread presence of scavenging pigs. The tests for hydatid disease were probably cross-reacting with proteins from this other tapeworm. If so, treating dogs would do no good.

We had hoped that the epidemiological studies would, through the sheer weight of evidence, persuade people to change their ways. The solutions were, on the face of it, obvious: have health inspectors at the slaughtering areas to cut out cysts and dispose of them properly; close in the slaughtering areas, and educate the public so that the dogs didn't get access to raw, cyst-infested meat; educate the public about hand washing after handling their dogs and about cleaning up dog feces to decrease fecal contamination of streets and houses; control the dog populations. Dominique prepared a video that was shown on TV. Dr. Joshi ran public education clinics and talked to members of the government about legislation. Yet after several years of hard work and good science, nothing seemed to have changed. Why not?

VIEWING THE HEAPS of animal parts and feces, the dogs and pigs and people foraging and defecating and washing up along the riverbank, I reconsidered previous attempts to "fix" problems of animal slaughtering, garbage, and disease transmission in Kathmandu. In the 1970s and 1980s, the Danish foreign aid agency built a large, modern abattoir (just like in Denmark!), the Germans built up the garbage disposal system (just like in Germany!), many countries helped train medical workers, and public health officials sneaked around at night dropping strychnine-laced pieces of meat for the street dogs (just as in Walt Disney's nightmares!) as a way to control rabies and hydatid disease.

In 1995, the Danish-built abattoir stood almost empty, the streets were again filling with garbage, well-trained medical workers were going back to their mountain villages to eke out a living from the barren soil, and the street dogs were doing just fine, fed and celebrated by members of the community.

These programs were based on good science and apparently sound logic. What was missing was any deep sense of culture: why did people behave in certain ways and not in others?

Scientific information is assumed to be objective and globally true, but that assumption is based on laboratory studies of basic phenomena. Can there be a science of place, one that explores phenomena that are locally true?

The earliest, most successful control program for echinococcosis was started in Iceland, where sheep rearing and sheepdogs go back many thousands of years and have long been an important part of cultural life. In 1869, Harald Krabbé, distressed at an overpopulation of dogs and the widespread distribution of "liver disease" associated with them, wrote a pamphlet in Icelandic explaining the life cycle of the disease. He then freely handed it out to every householder. Given the long, dark Icelandic winters, and the fact that this pamphlet was only the third document written in Icelandic (after the Bible and the Icelandic sagas), one can imagine that the idea of hydatid disease control became deeply ingrained in the Icelandic psyche. Even with that national breadth of understanding and a commitment to eradicate the disease (which included some drastic dog-control programs, such as legally forbidding dog ownership in the capital, Reykjavik), it took almost a hundred years for Iceland to get rid of the disease.

The success of the Icelanders emboldened many sheep-rearing countries to embark on similar control programs. The success of these programs has varied; even the most successful of them have depended on a well-educated population, regulated slaughtering facilities with veterinary health inspectors, and an attitude toward dogs that allowed for eradication of free-roaming dogs. In some cases, that success has depended on the degree to which Nepalese or Kenyans or Peruvians could be persuaded to behave like western Europeans or North Americans.

New Zealand's program was instructive; it began as a combination of education, dog registration, and provision of treatment drugs to dog owners. Education was directed at children in schools and at sheepdog owners, who were brought together to have their dogs treated with a purgative so that the feces could be examined for parasites. The program was much more successful among settlers of European descent than among the native Maori, for whom dogs played a different social role.

All of the successful hydatid disease control programs took decades to make progress and required a lot of public commitment and money. I wondered if it were even possible in Nepal.

One thing was clear: scientific work that tried to address issues that were policy-relevant, science for the public good, had to be embedded in a sense of social and ecological history. Budi Tamang, one of the Nepalese researchers on our team, recounted a story about a German development organization that went to Kirtipur, a city near Kathmandu, and installed a row of new toilets. The decision about where to place them and how to design them was most likely based on a proper scholarly assessment of public health needs in the community. For some reason, however, the people there wouldn't use the toilets. When asked, they told their benefactors, "Don't worry, maybe tomorrow we will use them." But they never did.

The Germans sent an anthropologist, who moved into the community, learned the Newari language, and joined the people's daily lives. This is what he found: During the unification of Nepal, the people of Kirtipur twice repelled the invading "unification" king. The third time, he approached from the west, although they expected him from the east. There followed a massacre. Since that time, the people of Kirtipur only defecate with their bums facing west, as an act of spite. The German toilets, as you might have guessed, were oriented so that the bums faced east. Once this mistake was rectified, the toilets were used.

Even such a simple thing as having a national act to regulate animal slaughtering—which Dr. Joshi had been working for years to get enacted—was stalled by political events. When our research team had started its work, Nepal was moving from a dictatorship to democracy. Many of the people we worked with were active in the pro-democracy movement. The political scene was exciting but chaotic. Every time the proposed act was near debate or about to be voted on, the government would collapse, new coalitions would form, and often new elections would be called. The chaotic emergence of democracy in Nepal (itself a good thing) was hindering another good thing, public health.

From a system of the king's rules, Nepal seemed to have moved rapidly to a system of no rules. Now when I bicycled around the crowded valley, I saw that the once-green rice fields of the valley were strewn with new, hastily erected, already-crumbling buildings. Everything was now for sale: intricately woven Tibetan carpets (made by Nepalese labor, polluting Nepalese water, using New Zealand wool and Indian dyes), gold and silver jewelry, turquoise and opal, Tibetan Buddhist artwork, fat laughing Buddhas and elephants from India, fierce Tibetan mastiffs, cuddly Lhasa apsos, and cheap imitations of Tibetan carpets. For the "alternative" tourists, there was the wilderness for sale: mountain climbing, white-water rafting, mountain vistas, cows, ducks, chickens, and dogs in the streets. There were also gambling casinos. In a sense, the romantic idea of a good-hearted and happy people of Nepal who worshipped strange, many-armed gods was also for sale as part of this exotic landscape.

This economic activity was bringing in a lot of money. In the best of all worlds, it would be translated into drinkable water, fresh air, and adequate food for the citizens of Nepal. But in Nepal, it was translated into impossible consumer demands and piles of garbage. How could the chaos be used as an opportunity to create something new? Many politicians, as well as the slaughterhouse owners and butchers, were responding to the demand for meat from tourists and the newly wealthy in this free-for-all economy. Could they be persuaded to reinvest in the health of their communities? How could we engage them in the work so that they would see its importance? My view of the relationship between science, policy, and public practice was shifting.

IN THE 1990S, several international networks of scholars were struggling with how to understand the complexity of the world we live in and to manage it, or adapt to it, in such ways that the human species could have a long and convivial sojourn on this planet. Among the ideas that emerged from one of these networks was that of ecosystem health. We talked about, measured, and promoted the health of individuals, families, and even cities. This being the case, could we not talk about the health of whole social-ecological systems?

I thought about the web of connections, as well as the facts, that our research had uncovered. They explained a lot about why some previous attempts to improve the well-being of the urban citizens in Kathmandu had been unsuccessful.

Family and cultural traditions of butchering perhaps once sustainable in sparsely populated rural areas were brought into the very different, more crowded urban setting of Kathmandu. Butchers didn't want to give up family traditions and become wage laborers in an animal-killing factory.

The economic, cultural, and family bases of human-dog relations, butchering practices, and the many dependent occupations of small-scale meat transporters and butcher shops throughout the city could not be altered simply by decreeing that it should be so or by making public health pronouncements. The street dogs were not only threats to public health but were also community police. Butchering and food hygiene practices depended not only on knowledge but also on the availability of clean water and affordable fuel for cooking, thus competing directly with economically powerful activities such as the carpet industry, which used—and wasted—huge amounts of water.

Even if the dogs could all be treated with an effective drug, it was not clear what the environmental consequences of the drug-in-feces would be. In the end, the communities involved would still be left with serious public health, economic, and environmental problems, many of which appeared to be considerably more pressing than this particular parasite. Of all the places these communities could spend what little spare cash they might have, why would they want to spend it on an antiparasitic drug or control program for dogs? Whatever would be done to respond to this parasite would have to be embedded in a much more comprehensive program of social transformation. If ecosystem health was a viable way of thinking about and working with complex public health problems, Kathmandu seemed to be an ideal case study.

At dusk, I sat nursing a beer on the roof terrace at the wonderful old Vajra Hotel, with its wood-carved walls, gardens, and traditional statuary, on the hillside up toward Swayambhunath, the Monkey Temple. I looked out over the darkening valley, the scattering of lights in this still-medieval city, the satellite dishes along the rooftops. The scent of dung and of wood fires and the clashing sounds of popular Indian and European music drifted up past me and into the cool, almost clean mountain air. If these new ideas about the health of social and ecological systems, combining community participation with systemic ecological understanding, could work here, they could work anywhere.

POSTSCRIPT

People often ask me what happened to hydatid disease in Kathmandu. I don't know, in part because it wasn't a priority for the citizens of wards 19 and 20. I do know, however, that the conditions that made it a problem have changed for the better.

In November 2001, we had the final workshop of a community-based ecosystem health project. Our research team this time included butchers, street sweepers, veterinarians, politicians, shop owners, anthropologists, and community activists.

Later, I took a picture of Dinesh Kadji, dynamic young chairman of the butchers' association, standing outside in the clean, sunlit courtyard beside the river. I told him that I thought there used to be an old water pump here. I had a picture of a woman taking water, with her children squatting around her, and, in the background, animals being slaughtered. It's right over there, he said, pointing to a clean, well-kept building across the yard, and he laughed.

The Dante-esque riverbanks I had first encountered in 1992 were transformed. Public parks with shrubs and trees and benches to sit on had been created next to the Bhimsentan Bridge. A man and a woman took care of new public toilets, as well as the gardens. The fees they charged were shared with the municipality. Although people were prohibited from defecating at the riverbank, I could see a fellow coming up out of the riverside grass, pulling up his pants. Still, it was much cleaner than it had been a decade previously. There were some piles of garbage, but many fewer than before. There were fewer dogs, as well. The trees were empty of vultures.

Next to the public parks, farther along the riverbank, were walls of tall grasses, and small private flower and vegetable gardens. Beyond that, rows of composting cow manure and stomach contents were aerated by plastic pipes, and flocks of ducks wandered among them, feasting on the larvae. To my right, away from the river, were cardboard and plastic recycling yards. A line of water buffalo were walking slowly along the street, followed by a lone herder. The herder guided them up a side street to a corrugated metal door. I slipped through the door after the animals. Around a brick courtyard were covered sheds. This was one of the twenty or so new, mid-scale slaughtering places scattered throughout wards 19 and 20. At a freshwater tap, women and children were pumping water into their brass pots and plastic pails.

Back outside, along the side streets, I came across the perpetually running stone taps. These taps are set in washing places below ground level for general community use and are maintained by traditional religious caretakers. Once filled with garbage, some of these washing places were now cleaned out and painted and were being used.

Since 2001, Nepal has been into and out of turmoil several times. In June 2001, Crown Prince Dipendra killed most of his family in a rage during a royal dinner, allegedly because his mother had disapproved of his choice for marriage. One uncle, Gyanendra Bir Bikram Shah, who was not at the meal, stepped up to the throne of this constitutional monarchy. Until he came to the throne, mainstream politicians had negotiated a delicate relationship with the Maoist party of Nepal and were bringing this rural insurgency group, fighting for economic development in the countryside, into the political process. When the new king came to power, this fragile peace fell apart.

In 2003 and 2004, as the Maoist war heated up, I became increasingly concerned that larger events could overwhelm a decade of good work and community learning. On the one hand, there had been a bomb near the Bhimsentan Bridge, where the young girl had once waited with her peaches, and the king had dissolved Parliament and received military aid from the U.S. to fight the "international terrorists," thus enabling him to back away from negotiated settlements. On the other hand, I received optimistic e-mails from one of our researchers, who was now heading a group in Nepal that builds on people's skills and strengths to achieve their hopes and dreams.

At one of our research workshops, the participants had been asked what stories they wanted their children to tell about them. What I hear from Dr. Joshi is that the communities are continuing their work, fighting for their democratic rights, creating stories of resilience in the midst of the battles among the tiresome capitalist, royalist, and Maoist ideologues. They have been monitoring water quality. Joshi himself is still running dog-vaccination clinics. The social-action Nepalese partners I worked with have mounted programs to improve the nutrition and health of the people in wards 19 and 20.

The people there have discovered the story they want their grandchildren to tell, and it is one of local democracy and commitment, of clean water and a thirst for knowledge and an impatience with systemic poverty and repression. I often think back to 1992 and remember the small girl on the bridge, waiting patiently with her lychees and peaches, and I hope she has a happy role in that story.

Shall We Tell Our Tales of Woe and Delight

. . .

WHAT DOES *it* ALL MEAN?

IS NATURE TELLING *us* SOMETHING?

IS IT *the* STORY WE WANT *to* TELL?

. . .

THE MEANING OF PULCHER'S OMEN

*H*UNDREDS OF diseases, most of which are not covered in this book, can be transmitted from other animals to people. Of 175 human diseases that are newly appearing or spreading to new areas of the world or to new populations (the so-called emerging diseases), 132 are considered zoonoses. Although the number of zoonotic diseases is large, the actual number of human cases, with a few exceptions, is very small. Nevertheless, given the massive volume of global trade and travel (both voluntary and forced, as with refugees) and the iniquitous inequities among the social conditions in which people around the world live, the possibility of catastrophic pandemics is not negligible. At one level, understanding how infections jump from other animals to people is not rocket science. They can be transferred through insects, environmental contamination, and direct contact, which includes situations where we rub noses with them as well as when they bite us, as in rabies, or we bite them, as in food.

Knowing how they are transmitted means that preventive measures are obvious, at least at the individual level. None of these measures are foolproof, but all of them are reasonably effective. Washing your hands with soap after handling animals or meat will take care of many bacteria and parasites; so-called antibacterial soaps are unnecessary and may only encourage the evolution of more aggressive microbial populations. Wearing a long-sleeved shirt outdoors and using insect repellents will help keep the mosquitoes and ticks in check. Cooking your food well will kill bacteria like *Salmonella* on the surface of—and parasites like *Toxoplasma* inside—your meat. Cleaning up dog poop and disposing of it by, say, composting, or in landfills, will help keep a variety of parasites and bacteria out of general circulation.

Even some preventive measures at the community level are straightforward and require only political will and some meager sense of global equity to share the necessary resources to implement them. Animal vaccination programs for rabies, anthrax, brucellosis, or avian influenza are all attainable with no major scientific discoveries. How to compost manure and dead animals, instead of burning or burying them, should be in the training manual for every person dealing with infectious diseases. Composting not only kills most bacteria and viruses but also generates useful fertilizer. Even developing a cheap, injectable reproductive control drug for male dogs should be relatively easy if any pharmaceutical company or funding agency could be persuaded to make it a priority. Cattle can be screened for various diseases such as sleeping sickness before being allowed into new, disease-free areas.

But the changing global patterns of zoonoses reflect not only individual behaviors. They are the result of complex social and ecological changes. Obvious examples of connections include those between the abandonment of farmland and Lyme disease, the economies of scale and avian influenza or salmonellosis, the degradation of wetlands and the piling up of old tires with water in them and mosquito-borne diseases, the love of raccoons (feeding them, shooting them) and rabies and parasites. At this systemic scale, we are faced with trade-offs. Abandonment of small farms may be seen as good (by some ecologists, for instance, or by some economists) or bad (by people who live in small communities). Hiking through the woods is both good for one's personal health (exercise, fresh air) and possibly risky (Lyme disease, West Nile). The dogs in Kathmandu were both community police and carriers of disease. At an international conference in 2006, a scientist from Turkey described how the killing of chickens to stop the spread of avian influenza resulted in outbreaks of tick-borne diseases in Turkish villages. The chickens had served as an important way of controlling ticks.

Resolving these complicated problems of emerging zoonoses in a more general sense comes down to rethinking our place in the world, how we think about progress, and how we do science. We, collectively as a species, are faced with fundamental questions of how we construct, evaluate, and use knowledge about the world around us.

If we look over the natural history of zoonoses and their emergence or re-emergence in the early twenty-first century, the general causes are a messy mixture of things. Often humans have created new urban or agricultural ecosystems in the ruins of older, non-human-dominated ecosystems. People have invaded new territories where other animals and their microbes have lived in some rough kind of harmony for millennia (Ebola, Marburg, Chagas disease). Other animals, such as rats, raccoons, and coyotes, have adapted to and changed human settlements, bringing with them viruses such as rabies and hantavirus, bacteria such as leptospirosis, and a variety of parasites. Economies of scale and monocultures in agriculture have created ideal conditions for the generation of epidemics of salmonellosis and avian influenza. Fast global travel and unfettered free trade have fostered the spread of epidemics. Loss of biodiversity, social inequity, marginalization of poor people, and the rapid sprawl of slums with bad housing, inadequate water, and standing sewage have created ecosystems that change the patterns of old infectious diseases and create opportunities for new ones. Climate change, much of it human induced, is contributing to the destabilization of ecosystems and the dispersal of animals and microbes into new areas. Talk of (re)creating natural harmony or ecological stability is an illusion.

Pulcher threw his sacred chickens overboard because he didn't like the message they were delivering. In some ways, the killing of millions of chickens in the face of H5N1 avian influenza virus is a similar act of defiance. A scientist—who is, if nothing else, a reader of omens—might ask why the chickens in Southeast Asia were becoming infected. One answer is that wild birds and livestock traders brought the virus to them. How did this happen? The draining of swamps and restructuring of landscapes for human use throughout the world has narrowed the options for wild birds to nest and to rest. Hence the birds are being forced into closer proximity to each other (more stress, more shedding of microbes) and to other species (more sharing of microbes and faster microbial evolution). They are also being channeled into smaller and fewer flight pathways, many of them close to expanding human settlements and agricultural enterprises.

Traders who are trucking and shipping poultry from place to place are responding to economic policies advocated by those in power. Those policies are put into place because urban dwellers want to eat more meat, and they want to pay less for it. The consequences of that trade for consumers are a cornucopia of low-cost meat at the grocery store and epidemics of food-borne diseases. The consequences of that trade for small farmers and for the rural social and ecological environment are loss of livelihoods, contaminated water, and loss of habitat for wildlife.

When viewed at this larger scale, the "whys" and "becauses" of any particular outbreak of, say, avian influenza, can go out in many different directions, with different winners and losers and feedback loops that are weakened (as between local farming practices and local environments) or created (as between local farming practices and global markets).

An outbreak on a particular chicken farm might be related to how the birds are housed, how crowded together they are, what other species live on the farms, what kinds of "bio-security" are available, and the structure of markets. This, in turn, has to do with urban demands for certain kinds of food, with economics and culture, and with who has power (both electrical, which is required to manage intensive poultry barns, and political, which is required to manage economic markets). The spread of an epidemic has to do with the technical capacity for diagnosis and response, with the value of fighting cocks and show birds, with education of poor people, and women in particular, with communication among those working with the health of people and other animals, and with drugs and hospitals available at the points where the epidemics start, which are often poor and marginalized.

In some ways, our understanding of the basic causes of infectious zoonotic diseases is not really new. In 1848, in a report to the Prussian government about an epidemic of typhus (carried by rat fleas) in Upper Silesia, biomedical scientist Rudolf Virchow suggested that what was needed was political reform and self-government, education, economic reform, agricultural reform (especially the development of co-operatives), road building, and a requirement that teachers and physicians speak the language of local people. The needs today have not changed all that much. We might add directives to protect and nurture healthy wetlands and woodlands, to put gardens on every flat rooftop, to refrain from building heat-enhancing freeways and parking lots, to shift away from personal cars to public transit, to clamp down on trade in "exotic" species, to regionalize agriculture, and to better manage international trade. These steps all are important and would be an excellent start, but they would be insufficient to address the fundamentals of social-ecological change and zoonotic disease emergence.

The rapidity and scale of changes associated with human activity now far exceed what we have seen before in our brief sojourn on this planet. We are sliding over the cusp of rapid climate change and environmental change. The speed and scope of change is what makes, say, direct genetic manipulation qualitatively different from cross-breeding, and the severe climate-change-associated droughts and floods and storms different from the droughts and storms and floods we have "always had." Some of the questions related to these rapid social-ecological systemic changes in the world cannot be answered using conventional laboratory-based science. Indeed, by taking these questions seriously, we are led to re-examine some of our fundamental notions of science and how it engages with the world. What is needed is a science capable of adapting quickly and interacting in real time with policy and management.

Our discovery of the world is a conversation between the preconceptions we have been taught (based on the perceptions of previous generations) and the perceptions we generate through our physical and mental experience of the exciting mess we live in. The sciences are a structured, systematic way of organizing our collective experiences and stories and testing and retesting them against new experiences. Science is by definition open and free to be challenged.

All of us look at the world through the windows of our eyes. We see trees and mountains, cars and ponies, children and a carpet stain for which the cat, we hope, was responsible. The windows we choose to look through reflect the questions we ask. This is true of scientists in North America as much as for poultry farmers in Indonesia. Biologists see not only wolves, dolphins, and fungi but also microbes that live all over our skin and threaten to invade our teeth.

Historically, we have often thought that the better the scientist, the smaller the window. This is why physicists, who see invisible little beings in the interstices of quirks and quarks, which through their strong and weak forces save us all from going dramatically to pieces, are considered the best scientists of all. They can take things that no one can see, even with a microscope, and that, like spirits, angels, and gods, can only be detected by their effects, and allow us to create things from them that could annihilate the earth. In this, they are the priests of the modern age. Any biologist who could develop a comprehensive physics of life would surely be in line for a Nobel Prize.

In many cases, the scientific questions have been formulated based on measures of importance decided by various funding agencies, or the scientists themselves, and have been answered based on the assumption "all other things being equal." The problem is, however, that for questions related to social and ecological change, all things are not equal, and many solutions to narrowly defined problems (how to produce more chickens with less labor input) add up to broadly defined, serious global problems (pandemics of chicken-related diseases). The synthesis and application of the many scientific facts generated by scientists has largely been left to non-scientists. Using little, manageable windows of observation, scientists have enabled human societies to treat sick people and animals, kill bacteria and fleas, rescue endangered species, prevent soil erosion, and increase business profitability. The systemic effects of solving all those problems as if they were not related to each other have been more species extinction, greater unemployment, widespread chemical contamination, and the emergence of new epidemics.

I recall how pleased I was when the vultures disappeared from the riverbanks in Kathmandu; the missing scavengers were at first a sign of success. Later I learned that vultures were dying all over the Indian subcontinent in huge numbers; in some places up to 97 percent of certain kinds of vultures had died. At first, investigators had thought it was some kind of viral epidemic. Then they discovered that a pain-killing drug, diclofenac, was being used in large doses throughout India to keep older cattle in comfort as they died. This in itself would seem to be a good and humane act. However, the vultures that fed on the carcasses of these cattle developed kidney failure and visceral gout (a buildup of uric acid); people recognized them by the way their heads drooped. The birds died soon after. The consequences of losing this major scavenger could be devastating, as semi-feral dogs congregate around rotting carcasses, spreading rabies and other diseases. Parsi, who place their dead in Towers of Death in Mumbai for the vultures to clean up, are wondering what will happen to their religious practices. I pondered whether the lack of vultures I had seen along the river in Kathmandu was a sign of success in controlling butchering activities or evidence of other feedback loops, the tragic consequences of the desire to keep cattle out of pain.

Most professionals and scientists, in the interests of efficiently and effectively solving different kinds of problems, are trained to see only certain things. Doctors see individual patients, public health workers see crowds and toilets, sociologists see a community of temples and roads, ecologists see a living, multifaceted community of communities, and many of us, increasingly, see just a big mess.

The world we live in *is* a complex mess that eludes even the best models scientists can devise. We experience it as a variety of colors and shapes that change over time, and from place to place, and from which we deduce functions, structures, and molecules interacting to form cells in organs in animals and plants, which interact with each other and the inanimate world to create the world we inhabit. Some complex systems theorists, mostly ecologists and sociologists, describe the world we live in as a series of nested hierarchies. As an individual, I have physical and social boundaries and an internal set of rules by which I function. I am also a member of a family with rules and boundaries, which is a member of various communities, each with its own rules and boundaries. By virtue of the fact that I eat, drink, perspire, breathe, urinate, and defecate, I can also be described according to my membership in several nested ecological systems.

The twentieth-century philosopher Arthur Koestler referred to each level in this hierarchy as a "holon," being both a whole and a part. The environmental scientist Henry Regier calls these nested hierarchies "holonocracies"; with its resonance of "democracy" and "autocracy," this term emphasizes the mutual power relationships and responsibilities. C.S. Holling and members of his Resilience Alliance use the term "panarchy," which can be traced back to the Belgian political scientist Paul Emile de Puydt in 1860. The alliance uses the term to emphasize the interplay between change and persistence across levels and over time.

Whatever term is used, these scientific theories provide useful frameworks for asking complicated questions about why zoonoses emerge and epidemics spread. Within these new ways of framing scientific query, scientists can begin to ask how draining a swamp today to prevent malaria or building a dam to prevent flooding might create spaces for new diseases, how one might begin to manage the trade-offs between hiking in the woods for good health and the possible exposure to Lyme disease or West Nile virus, and how trade to improve (some people's) livelihoods might create ideal conditions for pandemics.

Because the questions being asked bring together scientific inquiry with policy and action, answering them requires investigators to accommodate and evaluate multiple perspectives. The philosophers Silvio Funtowicz and Jerry Ravetz have called this publicly engaged science "post-normal." Going beyond "postmodern," in which many different viewpoints merely stand side by side, they propose that many different viewpoints need to be called upon to understand the world, define problems, and resolve issues in such a way as to sustain a convivial human existence on the earth.

As I have discovered in my own work in Nepal, Peru, Kenya, Uganda, Canada, and Cuba, resolution of complex problems requires good theory (complex systems theories have been very helpful here) and honest, risky social engagement. From this work has emerged a process for doing science (which I have described in my book *Ecosystem Sustainability and Health*). In this way of doing science, there are never any final, definitive experiments. This science is one of continual exploration and adaptation.

The collection of facts is not science. Science is the construction of the most compelling stories based on the best available evidence. Dinosaur bones without a story to explain them are just old bones. As scientists and as citizens, we need to open our field of vision and regain what many of science's earliest practitioners, like Pasteur and Virchow, had—the hunter's habit of peripheral vision, seeing the slight movement in the trees to our left, the slow rising of a grass stem brushed against in the moment before our arrival, the intuition of being-in-the-world.

The challenge for scientists and non-scientists alike is to find ways to listen to, and to respect, each other. Stories about fighting cocks and their value in Thai society and of bird migrations and of poor farmers selling chickens so that their children can attend school are as relevant to this kind of science, and to the prevention of a pandemic, as are stories of viral structure and evolution.

The old patriarchal we-are-right-and-you-are-wrong stories are over. At a global level, the old stories ended in the sighing heave of rubble and, through the gritty air, the inchoate wailing of sirens, and the harsh, misanthropic snarl of preaching. They are finished. The End. What can they now tell us? Their grand visions can't help us anymore. If we stick to them, we will awake in the morning with our collective heads cut off, and the world will go on without us. And yet, we live by stories, and we need some sense of a global story if we want to promote global solidarity and a healthy planet.

In *1001 Arabian Nights*, Sultan Schahriar feels betrayed by his first wife. He seeks his revenge on women in general by having his grand vizier present him with a fresh bride every night and then having her strangled (by the grand vizier) the next morning. Scheherazade, beautiful daughter of the grand vizier, decides to put herself on the line for the sake of all women. In a successful, non-violent stratagem, she recruits her less-than-beautiful sister, Dinarzade. Every day, just before dawn, her sister awakens her and asks Scheherazade to tell her a story. The sultan is, of course, listening in and is left at dawn wanting to hear more. Every day, the sultan decides to spare her, and eventually he falls in love, first with Scheherazade's stories and then with her; he abandons his brutal, tyrannical, obsessive plans. She lives a long and meaningful life and is celebrated by young people and peace activists the world over.

The tale of Scheherazade is, finally, a tale about all of us. The earth, like Schahriar, has cut the heads off many species before us. Global history is replete with sudden or slow mass extinctions. The earth is literally built from the bones and decomposed molecules of our forbears. We humans, too, have betrayed our hosts and the bacteria who collaborated to make us possible. If we are not soon to go the way of the glyptodont and the pterosaur, then our global human family needs a good dose of psychotherapy—not just any therapy, but a narrative therapy in which we have reimagined and retold our tale as one of survival, justice, ecological at-home-ness, and conviviality. To find this story requires a (re)search effort beyond anything we have tried before; like Scheherazade, our lives depend on it.

Some people would argue that the new human story is simply a grand imagining told by evolutionary biologists and ecologists, some version of Darwin (evolution), Watson and Crick (DNA), or E.O. Wilson (sociobiology). The ways of science have taught us much. We have a much richer understanding of the universe than we had, say, one hundred years ago. But science as we have known it has also reached a kind of end, a Sisyphean conundrum in which we are unveiling the vast, swampy realms of our ignorance faster than we are able to fashion little boardwalks of knowledge to support our daily steps. It turns out that controlling some of the great infectious-disease scourges of human development—smallpox, tuberculosis, and the plague—was the easy part of doing medical and health science. Now we have to find ways to live in some sort of uneasy balance with the remaining tumult of plant, animal, and microbial life of which the world is composed.

The outbreaks and epidemics of zoonoses globally can be explained by bringing together the mass of data collected on these subjects over several decades and telling a story of hunger, technological optimism, cheap oil prices, the economics of scale, obsessions with personal health, and economic inequity. Without that story, any preventive strategies will be a mere floundering around in the muddy data and, more often than not, will make the long-term problems worse rather than better. I am not advocating a retreat into superstitions or unsubstantiated stories, nor do I have much patience for the view—preached by some among the so-called climate change skeptics—that because the world is complex and the outcomes of our actions are uncertain, we should do nothing. Not all stories are equal, and science has indeed added a new element, an essential element, to how we assess quality, how we discover and live our emergent story.

A story rings false, proves itself weak, inadequate to the task of helping us find our collective way through a mysterious universe, if it must rely on brute force to "prove" its veracity. To the extent that Christianity, Islam, Buddhism, state capitalism (as practiced by Stalin), corporate capitalism, and institutional science rely on bombs, planes crashing into tall buildings, assassinations, armies, popes, excommunications, shunnings, invasions, old boys, and patents, they simple prove their own weakness. At the same time, to the extent that the proponents of religions and ideologies tell their stories freely and openly, vulnerable to challenge, and modify them in the face of new observations, they contribute to the emerging story of the becoming universe.

For a story to prove its quality, both the means of observation and the observations themselves must be transparent and open to challenge and counter-challenge. This is the great contribution of science, which previous stories did not have: in science, there is no pope, no imam, no patented or non-publicly available information, no creed agreed upon by a bunch of well-meaning or power-hungry old men (pick your conspiracy), no canon of accepted truth that trumps careful observation and experience. This is the good news we need to whisper abroad, to take back into the real world, democratizing science, democratizing religion and ideology, so that we all become scholars and priests and scientists. But not just any kind of scientists.

The main character in William Boyd's novel *Armadillo* is searching for a word to signify the opposite of serendipity. "Serendipity" is derived from Serendip, an earlier name for what is now Sri Lanka. Heroes in an old Persian folktale had the faculty of making happy and unexpected discoveries by accident. Boyd suggests that a term to mean the opposite of "serendipity" be based on a fictional country that is cold and barren, called Zembla. Thus, "zemblanity" would be "the faculty of making unhappy, unlucky and expected discoveries by design."

This faculty is certainly what characterizes the disciplines I work in—epidemiology, environmental and biomedical sciences. We think some things such as feces in water or diesel fumes in air or smoking cigarettes might cause people and animals to get sick, so we set up studies to prove that this is so. To the surprise of no one except those who are making money by dumping this stuff into our air and water, we find they do cause disease. Much global monitoring of disease and environmental degradation is also characterized by zemblanity. But the problems of the twenty-first century are unpredictable, uncertain; they will continue to surprise us. We, as a species, need to find solutions, ways of adapting to unexpected changes of ecosystems and economies, rather than simply documenting problems. To do this, we need a new serendipitous science, a post-normal science, a science that is not afraid to look at everything, to accommodate uncertainty, mystery, struggles for justice, and to admit storytelling into its campfire circle.

All of us, as global citizens, must become Scheherazade, the beautiful storyteller, and Dinarzade, the one who elicits this insurrection of marginalized stories from all over the world. These stories are not just of people but also of every living thing and of the earth itself. The stories in this book have been about diseases, diseases that like Pulcher's chickens are a voice, a reminder, a calling. The agents that cause disease in people and other animals and plants are thriving communities of tiny living beings; diseases are the consoling and horrific reminder that we are not alone, that our story has many voices, and that sometimes, if we ignore them, the tiniest of voices will inhabit our bodies and speak to us of mysteries we have ignored.

. We, the people, are a gift from nature that she will take back to herself when we die and the microbes recycle us. Bringing together our best political, religious, ecological, evolutionary, and philosophical stories with the artifacts we unearth through our best scholarly investigations, it is our work to jostle and sing and shout and whisper them into something greater than the sum of the data, a multilayered, multiperson, multiethnic, multispecies tale of life on this planet.

Claudius Pulcher no doubt lost his battle at Drepana in 249 BC as the result of the usual mix of bad timing and poor maritime skills. Still, one wonders about the sacred chickens that refused to eat. We don't have to believe that birds are omens, as part of some complicated spiritual mathematics, for us to take home important messages. If I were to articulate what I think Pulcher's Omen is, it is this: that all natural events tell us something well beyond the immediate causes we identify, and that if we observe carefully, we might yet survive another millennium here.

The natural history of zoonoses tells us that our struggle with infectious diseases is not a war—or, if it is, it is a war against ourselves. The microbes are all around us, in us, and in our animal companions on this planet. Our struggle must ultimately be one of global solidarity and keen, careful ecological awareness. We must, above all, *care*. Circling the wagons and stockpiling drugs and vaccines in Ottawa, Washington, and Geneva will not solve this problem. We must dig into our history, rediscovering the roots of what it means to be human. The very ancient Indo-European word for "earth," *dhghem*, gave us not only the word "human" but also the word "humus," the organic component of soil created by bacteria, as well as the words "humble" and "humane."

In this new task, we are all observing the world, collectively, as if for the first time, and constructing meaning from it. In the age of gun-toting peace-makers, God-fearing hell-raisers, and utopian pillagers, at a time when all the previous global stories have brought us rack and ruin, this is no small task. The good news is that, community by community, the world over, a novel global vision is emerging, revealing a planet full of complexity and mystery and beauty we never suspected was there, a world unexplored because we lacked the theoretical and practical tools. From this novel vision is emerging a global novel, full of stories, intriguing and wonderful tales hiding in the shadows of our grand delusions. The biosphere might yet spare us. Or, if the stories don't save us, they will at least, on our deathbed, in the last days of our species, have us saying, "We did quite all right, didn't we? We left a story of ourselves worth telling the universe."

SELECTED READINGS

Acha, P.N., and B. Szyfres. 2003. *Zoonoses and Communicable Diseases Common to Man and Animals.* 2nd ed. Washington, D.C.: Pan American Health Organization.

Brock, Arthur J., ed. and ann. 1972. *Greek Medicine: Being Extracts Illustrative of Medical Writers from Hippocrates to Galen.* New York: AMS Press.

Burnet, Sir M., and White, D.O. 1972. *Natural History of Infectious Disease.* Cambridge: Cambridge University Press.

Brothwell, D., and A.T. Sandison, eds. 1967. *Diseases in Antiquity: A Survey of the Diseases, Injuries and Surgery in Early Populations.* Springfield, IL: Charles C. Thomas.

Charron, D., D. Waltner-Toews, A. Maarouf, and M.A. Stalker. 2003. A Synopsis of Known and Potential Diseases and Parasites of Humans and Animals Associated with Climate Change in Ontario. *A Synopsis of Known and Potential Diseases Associated with Climate Change,* Ontario Forest Research Information Paper no. 154. S. Greitenhagen, and T.L. Noland (comps.). Sault Ste. Marie, ON: Ontario Forest Research Institute, Ontario Ministry of Natural Resources.

Clutton-Brock, Juliet. 1981. *Domesticated Animals from Early Times.* London: Heinemann, British Museum (Natural History).

——. *A Natural History of Domesticated Mammals.* 2nd ed. Cambridge: Cambridge University Press.

Committee on the Applications of Ecological Theory to Environmental Problems, Commission on Life Sciences, National Research Council. 1986. *Ecological Knowledge and Environmental Problem-Solving: Concepts and Case Studies.* Washington, D.C.: National Academy Press.

Corvalan, C., S. Hales, and A.J. McMichael, eds. 2005. *Ecosystems and Human Well-Being Synthesis.* Geneva: WHO.

Desowitz, Robert S. 1981. *New Guinea Tapeworms and Jewish Grandmothers: Tales of Parasites and People.* New York: Avon Books.

Evans, R.G., M.L. Barer, and T.R. Marmor. 1994. *Why Are Some People Healthy and Others Not?* New York: Aldine de Gruyter.

Fiennes, Richard N. 1978. *Zoonoses and the Origins and Ecology of Human Disease.* London: Academic Press.

Garrett, Laurie. 1994. *The Coming Plague.* New York: Penguin Books.

Hyams, Edward. 1972. *Animals in the Service of Man: 10,000 Years of Domestication.* London: J.M. Dent & Sons.

Institute of Medicine. 1992. *Emerging Infections: Microbial Threatsto Health in the United States.* Washington, D.C.: National Academy Press.

Krauss, Hartmut, Albert Weber, Max Appel, Burkhard Enders, Henry D. Isenberg, Hans Gerd Schiefer, Werner Slenczka, Alexander von Graevenitz, and Horst Zahner. 2003. *Zoonoses: Infectious Diseases Transmissible from Animals to Humans.* 3rd ed. Washington, D.C.: ASM Press.

Margulis, Lynn, and Dorion Sagan. 1986. *Microcosmos: Four Billion Years of Evolution from Our Microbial Ancestors.* New York: Summit Books.

Marrie, Thomas, ed. 1990. *Q Fever, Volume 1: The Disease.* Boca Raton: CRC Press.

McMichael, A.J. 1993. *Planetary Overload: Global Environmental Change and the Health of the Human Species.* Cambridge: Cambridge University Press.

McNeill, W.H. *Plagues and Peoples.* 1976. Garden City, NY: Anchor Books.

Palmer, S.R., Lord Soulsby, and D.I.H. Simpson. 1998. *Zoonoses: Biology, Clinical Practice and Public Health Control.* Oxford: Oxford University Press.

Pavlovsky, E.N. 1966. *Natural Nidality of Transmissible Diseases; With Special Reference to the Landscape Ecology of Zooanthroponoses.* English trans. F.K. Plous Jr. Urbana, IL: University of Illinois Press.

Scheld, W.M., William Craig, and James Hughes, eds. 1998. *Emerging Infections,* vols. 1 & 2. Washington, D.C.: ASM Press.

Schwabe, C.W. 1984. *Veterinary Medicine and Human Health.* Baltimore: Williams & Wilkins.

Scullard, Howard H. 1960. *A History of the Roman World from 753 to 146 BC.* 3rd ed. London: Methuen.

Tarán, L., ed. *Aristotle, On the Parts of Animals.* Greek and Roman Philosophy, vol. 26. New York: Garland Publishing.

Waltner-Toews, David. 2004. *Ecosystem Sustainability and Health: A Practical Approach.* Cambridge: Cambridge University Press.

——. 2007. *Food, Sex and Salmonella.* 2nd ed. Vancouver: Greystone Books.

Waltner-Toews, D., and A. Ellis. 1992. *Good For Your Animals, Good For You.* Guelph, ON: Pet Trust.

Zinsser, Hans. 1971 (8th printing of Bantam edition). *Rats, Lice and History.* Boston: Little, Brown.

OTHER SOURCES

The history, characterization, and re-emergence of zoonoses are addressed in a wide variety of scientific journals and technical reports, and I have searched most of them over the past decades for material for teaching and research. Two journals that have emerged since the 1990s deserve special mention. *Emerging Infectious Diseases* is published by the National Center for Infectious Diseases, United States Centers for Disease Control and Prevention, and is available free online. *EcoHealth*, which addresses relationships between human health, animal health, and ecosystem sustainability, is the official journal of the International Society for Ecology and Health and is published by Springer. A good ongoing source of information for zoonotic diseases is also ProMED, an online reporting system for health professionals working with infectious disease. It can be found at www.promedmail.org.

Information on global environmental change and its impacts on human well-being can be found at the Web site for the Millennium Ecosystem Assessment at http://www.maweb.org.

ACKNOWLEDGMENTS

*I*T IS A CLICHÉ, but so many people have contributed to my knowledge and understanding of zoonoses that it would be impossible to list them all, and in trying (which, of course, I will), I will forget some. Sorry. Chalk it up to a "George Bush" moment. The graduate students I have worked with over the years have educated me far more than they know. I have mentioned some of them in the text as it was relevant, but they include: James Valcour, Cynthia Neudoerffer, Sandra LeFebvre, Lea Berrang, Karen Morrison, Katarina Pintar, Sharon Calvin, Kate Thomas, Popy Dimoulas, Jennifer Goy, Andria Jones, Thomas Gitau, Pia Muchaal, Dominique Charron, Nirmala Budhram, Erin Sifton, Simon Ferrazzi, Marieke Wevers-Carroll, John VanLeeuwen, Siti Ramanoon, Tamsyn Rowley, Bambang Sumiarto, Dominique Baronet, Andrea Ellis, Chow Ka-Wai, Maria Donado, Parminder Raina, Cord Heuer, Ingrid Vanderlinden, John Campbell, Michael Heald, and my post-doc during the TriCouncil Eco-Research project, Ellen Wall.

Thanks to my friends and colleagues in the Ecosystems, Climate Change and Health Omnibus (ECCHO), EcoHealth, and zoonoses worlds, including, in no particular order, Craig

Stephen, Margot Parkes, Bruce Wilcox, Ole Nielsen, Carl Ribble, Scott McEwen, Peter Daszak, Alonso Aguirre, Pierre Horwitz, Ian Barker, Bruce Hunter, John McDermott, Barry Smit, Robbin Lindsay, Nick Ogden, Abdel Maarouf, Martin Bunch, Dean Bavington, Wendelin Galatianos, and Manon D. Fleury. And members of the Dirk Gently Gang and its hangers-on, especially Silvio Funtwicz, Jerry Ravetz, Gilberto Gallopin, Ernesto Raez-Luna, Tim Allen, and the late, greatly missed James Kay. Thanks to the many students who took my graduate course in Epidemiology of Zoonoses and kept pushing me to the edge of new knowledge. Special thanks to my readers Sandy LeFebvre, Craig Stephen, and Kathy Waltner-Toews for their timely feedback on various chapters.

Thanks to Nancy Flight, the diligent editor at Greystone who helped me to find my voice in the cacophony of stories trying to get out of my head, and to Wendy Fitzgibbons, for her attention to detail.

And finally, thanks to Carolyn Swayze, my agent, for thinking I could do this, and then getting me a contract so that I had to.

INDEX